Praise for *Brain on Fire*

"The best reporters never stop asking questions, and Cahalan is no exception . . . The result is a kind of anti-memoir, an out-of-body personal account of a young woman's fight to survive one of the cruelest diseases imaginable. And on every level, it's remarkable. . . . Cahalan is nothing if not tenacious, and she perfectly tempers her brutal honesty with compassion and something like vulnerability. It's indisputable that Cahalan is a gifted reporter, and *Brain on Fire* is a stunningly brave book. But even more than that, she's a naturally talented prose stylist—whip-smart but always unpretentious—and it's nearly impossible to stop reading her, even in the book's most painful passages. . . . *Brain on Fire* comes from a place of intense pain and unthinkable isolation, but finds redemption in Cahalan's unflagging, defiant toughness. It's an unexpected gift of a book from one of America's most courageous young journalists."

—NPR

"A fascinating look at the disease that—if not for a nick-of-time diagnosis—could have cost this vibrant, vital young woman her life."

—*People*

"A young *New York Post* reporter contracts a rare brain disorder, recovers against the odds, then puts her restored mind to use investigating the disease's medical underpinnings. . . . Swift and haunting."

—*Scientific American*

"A dramatic and suspenseful book that draws you into her story and holds you there until the last page . . . I recommend it highly."

—*The Lancet*

"What is most impressive about *Brain on Fire* is that Cahalan has little recollection of her month of insanity. . . . Thanks partially to her talent as a journalist and to the fact that her parents kept journals, Cahalan was able to recapture her month, leaving no holes in the narrative."

—*The Daily Texan*

"With eagle-eyed precision and brutal honesty, Susannah Cahalan turns her journalistic gaze on herself as she bravely looks back on one of the most harrowing and unimaginable experiences one could ever face: the loss of mind, body, and self. *Brain on Fire* is a mesmerizing story of a promising young writer's rapid descent into madness, due to a mysterious and debilitating disease. But thanks to a dedicated doctor and the undying love and devotion of her family and boyfriend, she returns to the world she left behind wiser, stronger, and very much alive."

—Mira Bartók, *New York Times* bestselling author of
The Memory Place

"*Brain on Fire* is a swift, engrossing read and, unquestionably, an important book on both a human and a medical level. Cahalan's elegantly written memoir of her dramatic descent into madness opens up discussion of the cutting-edge neuroscience behind a disease that may affect thousands of people around the world, and it offers powerful insight into the subjective workings of our minds."

—Mehmet Oz, M.D., professor and vice chair, Department of
Surgery, New York Presbyterian-Columbia Medical Center

"Susannah Cahalan describes in chilling detail her descent into an inexplicable madness. So vivid and honest is Cahalan's portrayal that the reader is drawn inexorably into her world as it disintegrates until she loses her very self—emotionally, physically and mentally . . . It is a story of everyday heroes—her family, friends, and the determined doctors who steadfastly fought for her . . . Bravo to Ms. Cahalan who has been to hell and back and chronicles her journey so poignantly that we all may benefit."

—Barbara Arrowsmith-Young, author of
The Woman Who Changed Her Brain

BRAIN
ON
FIRE

MY MONTH OF MADNESS

SUSANNAH CAHALAN

SIMON & SCHUSTER PAPERBACKS
New York   London   Toronto   Sydney   New Delhi

SIMON & SCHUSTER PAPERBACKS
An Imprint of Simon & Schuster, Inc.
1230 Avenue of the Americas
New York, NY 10020

A note to readers: Names and identifying details of some of the people
portrayed in this book have been changed.

This Simon & Schuster trade paperback edition July 2018

For information about special discounts for bulk purchases, please contact
Simon & Schuster Special Sales at 1-866-506-1949 or
business@simonandschuster.com.

The Simon & Schuster Speakers Bureau can bring authors to your live event.
For more information or to book an event contact the Simon & Schuster Speakers
Bureau at 1-866-248-3049 or visit our website at www.simonspeakers.com.

Designed by Mspace/Maura Fadden Rosenthal

"Intake Interview" from WHEELING MOTEL by Franz Wright, copyright © 2009 by
Franz Wright. Used by permission of Alfred A. Knopf, a division of Random House, Inc.

"California Dreamin'"
Words and Music by John Phillips and Michelle Phillips.
Copyright © 1965 UNIVERSAL MUSIC CORP.
Copyright Renewed.
All Rights Reserved. Used by Permission.
Reprinted by Permission of Hal Leonard Corporation.

Manufactured in the United States of America

10 9 8 7 6 5 4 3 2 1

The Library of Congress has cataloged the hardcover edition as follows:
Cahalan, Susannah.
Brain on fire: my month of madness / Susannah Cahalan.
p. cm.
1. Cahalan, Susannah—Health. 2. Cahalan, Susannah—Mental health. 3. Encephalitis—Patients—United States—Biography. 4. Autoimmune diseases—Patients—United
States—Biography. 5. Frontal lobes—Diseases—Patients—United States—Biography.
6. Limbic system—Diseases—Patients—United States—Biography. 7. Diagnostic
errors—United States—Case studies. I. Title.
RC390.C24 2012
616.8'320092—dc23   2012012670

ISBN 978-1-9821-0948-6
ISBN 978-1-4516-2139-6 (ebook)

Dedicated to those without a diagnosis

CONTENTS

PART THREE: IN SEARCH OF LOST TIME

AUTHOR'S NOTE

The existence of forgetting has never been proved: we only know that some things do not come to our mind when we want them to.

—FRIEDRICH NIETZSCHE

Because of the nature of my illness, and its effect on my brain, I remember only flashes of actual events, and brief but vivid hallucinations, from the months in which this story takes place. The vast majority of that time remains blank or capriciously hazy. Because I am physically incapable of remembering that time, writing this book has been an exercise in my comprehending what was lost. Using the skills I've learned as a journalist, I've made use of the evidence available—hundreds of interviews with doctors, nurses, friends, and family; thousands of pages of medical records; my father's journal from this period; the hospital notebook that my divorced parents used to communicate with each other; snippets of video footage of me taken by hospital cameras during my stay; and notebooks upon notebooks of recollections, consultations, and impressions—to help me re-create this evasive past. I have changed some names and defining characteristics, but otherwise this is wholly a work of nonfiction, a blend of memoir and reportage.

Even still, I readily admit that I'm an unreliable source. No matter how much research I've done, the consciousness that defines me as a person wasn't present then. Plus, I'm biased. It's my life, and so at the core of this story is the old problem of journalism, made a hundredfold messier. There are undoubtedly things that I have gotten wrong, mysteries I will never solve, and many moments left forgotten and unwritten. What is left, then, is a journalist's inquiry into that deepest part of the self—personality, memory, identity— in an attempt to pick up and understand the pieces left behind.

*A*t first, there's just darkness and silence.
"Are my eyes open? Hello?"

I can't tell if I'm moving my mouth or if there's even anyone to ask. It's too dark to see. I blink once, twice, three times. There is a dull foreboding in the pit of my stomach. That, I recognize. My thoughts translate only slowly into language, as if emerging from a pot of molasses. Word by word the questions come: Where am I? Why does my scalp itch? Where is everyone? Then the world around me comes gradually into view, beginning as a pinhole, its diameter steadily expanding. Objects emerge from the murk and sharpen into focus. After a moment I recognize them: TV, curtain, bed.

I know immediately that I need to get out of here. I lurch forward, but something snaps against me. My fingers find a thick mesh vest at my waist holding me to the bed like a—what's the word?—straitjacket. The vest connects to two cold metal side rails. I wrap my hands around the rails and pull up, but again the straps dig into my chest, yielding only a few inches. There's an unopened window to my right that looks onto a street. Cars, yellow cars. Taxis. I am in New York. Home.

Before the relief finishes washing over me, though, I see her. The purple lady. She is staring at me.

"Help!" I shout. Her expression never changes, as if I hadn't said a thing. I shove myself against the straps again.

"Don't you go doing that," she croons in a familiar Jamaican accent.

"Sybil?" But it couldn't be. Sybil was my childhood babysitter. I haven't seen her since I was a child. Why would she choose today to reenter my life? "Sybil? Where am I?"

"The hospital. You better calm down." It's not Sybil.

"It hurts."

The purple lady moves closer, her breasts brushing against my *face as she bends across me to unhook the restraints, starting on the right and moving to the left. With my arms free, I instinctually raise my right hand to scratch my head. But instead of hair and scalp, I find a cotton hat. I rip it off, suddenly angry, and raise both hands to inspect my head further. I feel rows and rows of plastic wires. I pluck one out—which makes my scalp sting—and lower it to eye level; it's pink. On my wrist is an orange plastic band. I squint, unable to focus on the words, but after a few seconds, the block letters sharpen: FLIGHT RISK.*

I have felt that odd whirr of wings in the head.
—VIRGINIA WOOLF, *A Writer's Diary:*
Being Extracts from the Diary of Virginia Woolf

CHAPTER 1

BEDBUG BLUES

Maybe it all began with a bug bite, from a bedbug that didn't exist.

One morning, I'd woken up to find two red dots on the main purplish-blue vein running down my left arm. It was early 2009, and New York City was awash in bedbug scares: they infested offices, clothing stores, movie theaters, and park benches. Though I wasn't naturally a worrier, my dreams had been occupied for two nights straight by finger-long bedbugs. It was a reasonable concern, though after carefully scouring the apartment, I couldn't find a single bug or any evidence of their presence. Except those two bites. I even called in an exterminator to check out my apartment, an overworked Hispanic man who combed the whole place, lifting up my sofa bed and shining a flashlight into places I had never before thought to clean. He proclaimed my studio bug free. That seemed unlikely, so I asked for a follow-up appointment for him to spray. To his credit, he urged me to wait before shelling out an astronomical sum to do battle against what he seemed to think was an imaginary infestation. But I pressed him to do it, convinced that my apartment, my bed, my *body* had been overrun by bugs. He agreed to return and exterminate.

Concerned as I was, I tried to conceal my growing unease from my coworkers. Understandably, no one wanted to be associated with a person with a bedbug problem. So at work the following day, I walked as nonchalantly as possible through the newsroom of the *New York Post* to my cubicle. I was careful to conceal my bites and tried to appear casual, normal. Not that "normal" means a lot at the *Post*.

3

Though it's notoriously obsessed with what's new, the *Post* is nearly as old as the nation itself. Established by Alexander Hamilton in 1801, it is the longest continually run newspaper in the country. In its first century alone, the paper crusaded for the abolition movement and helped promote the creation of Central Park. Today the newsroom itself is cavernous yet airless, filled with rows of open cubicles and a glut of filing cabinets packed with decades of unused, forgotten documents. The walls are freckled with clocks that don't run, dead flowers hung upside down to dry, a picture of a monkey riding a border collie, and a big foam Six Flags finger, all memorabilia from reporters' assignments. The PCs are ancient, the copy machines the size of small ponies. A small utility closet that once served as a smoking room now holds supplies, and is marked by a weathered sign warning that the smoking room no longer exists, as if someone might accidentally wander in for a cigarette among the monitors and video equipment. This has been my eccentric little world for the past seven years, since I started here as a seventeen-year-old intern.

Especially around deadline, the room buzzes with activity—keyboards clacking, editors yelling, reporters cackling—the perfect stereotype of a tabloid newsroom.

"Where's the fucking picture to go with this caption?"

"How is it that he didn't know she was a prostitute?"

"What color were the socks of the guy who jumped off the bridge?"

It's like a bar without alcohol, filled with adrenaline-soaked news junkies. The cast of characters here is unique to the *Post*: the brightest headline writers in the business, the hardened newshounds hunting after exclusives, and type-A workaholics who possess the chameleon ability to either befriend or antagonize almost anyone. Still, on most days, the newsroom is subdued, as everyone silently combs through court documents, interviews sources, or reads newspapers. Often, like today, the newsroom is as quiet as a morgue.

Heading toward my desk to start the day, I wove through the rows of cubicles marked by green Manhattan street signs: Liberty

Street, Nassau Street, Pine Street, and William Street, throwbacks to a time when the *Post* was actually flanked by those downtown streets in its previous home at the South Street Seaport. My desk is at Pine Street. Amid the silence, I slid into my seat beside Angela, my closest friend at the paper, and gave her a tense smile. Trying not to let my question echo too loudly across the noiseless room, I asked, "You know anything about bedbug bites?"

I often joked that if I ever had a daughter, I'd want her to be like Angela. In many ways, she is my newsroom hero. When I first met her, three years before, she was a soft-spoken, shy young woman from Queens, only a few years older than me. She had arrived at the *Post* from a small weekly paper and since then had matured under the pressure of a big-city tabloid into one of the *Post*'s most talented reporters, churning out reams of our best stories. Most late Friday nights, you'd find Angela writing four stories on split screens simultaneously. I couldn't help but look up to her. Now I really needed her advice.

Hearing that dreaded word, *bedbugs*, Angela scooted her chair away from mine. "Don't tell me you have them," she said with an impish smile. I started to show her my arm, but before I could get into my tale of woe, my phone rang.

"You ready?" It was the new Sunday editor, Steve. He was just barely in his midthirties, yet he had already been named head editor of the Sunday paper, the section I worked for, and despite his friendliness, he intimidated me. Every Tuesday, each reporter had a pitch meeting to showcase some of his or her ideas for that Sunday's paper. At the sound of his voice, I realized with panic that I was completely unprepared for this week's meeting. Usually I had at least three coherent ideas to pitch; they weren't always great, but I always had something. Now I had nothing, not even enough to bluff my way through the next five minutes. How had I let that happen? This meeting was impossible to forget, a weekly ritual that we all fastidiously prepared for, even during days off.

Bedbugs forgotten, I widened my eyes at Angela as I stood back up, gamely hoping it all would work out once I got to Steve's office.

Nervously, I walked back down "Pine Street" and into Steve's office. I sat down next to Paul, the Sunday news editor and close friend who had mentored me since I was a sophomore in college, giving him a nod but avoiding direct eye contact. I readjusted my scratched-up wide-framed *Annie Hall* glasses, which a publicist friend once described as my own form of birth control because "no one will sleep with you with those on."

We sat there in silence for a moment, as I tried to let myself be comforted by Paul's familiar, larger-than-life presence. With his shock of prematurely white hair and his propensity to toss the word *fuck* around like a preposition, he is the essence of a throw-back newsman and a brilliant editor.

He had given me a shot as a reporter during the summer of my sophomore year of college after a family friend introduced us. After a few years in which I worked as a runner, covering breaking news and feeding information to another reporter to write the piece, Paul offered me my first big assignment: an article on the debauchery at a New York University fraternity house. When I returned with a story and pictures of me playing beer pong, he was impressed with my chutzpah; even though the exposé never ran, he assigned me more stories until I had been hired on full time in 2008. Now, as I sat in Steve's office wholly unprepared, I couldn't help but feel like a work in progress, not worthy of Paul's faith and respect.

The silence deepened until I looked up. Steve and Paul were staring at me expectantly, so I just started talking, hoping something would come. "I saw this story on a blog . . . ," I said, desperately plucking up wisps of half-formed ideas.

"That's really just not good enough," Steve interrupted. "You need to be bringing in better stuff than this. Okay? Please don't come in with nothing again." Paul nodded, his face blazing red. For the first time since I'd started working on my high school newspaper, journalism disagreed with me. I left the meeting furious at myself and bewildered by my own ineptitude.

"You okay?" Angela asked as I returned to my desk.

"Yeah, you know, I'm just bad at my job. No big deal," I joked grimly.

She laughed, revealing a few charmingly crooked incisor teeth. "Oh, come on, Susannah. What happened? Don't take it seriously. You're a pro."

"Thanks, Ang," I said, sipping my lukewarm coffee. "Things just aren't going my way."

I brooded over the day's disasters that evening as I walked west from the News Corp. building on Sixth Avenue, through the tourist clusterfuck that is Times Square, toward my apartment in Hell's Kitchen. As if purposely living the cliché of a New York writer, I rented a cramped one-room studio, where I slept on a pullout sofa. The apartment, eerily quiet, overlooked the courtyard of several tenements, and I often awoke not to police sirens and grumbling garbage trucks but to the sound of a neighbor playing the accordion on his balcony.

Still obsessed with my bites, despite the exterminator's assurance that I had nothing to worry about, I prepared for him to spray the place and spent that night discarding things that could be harboring bedbugs. Into the garbage went my beloved *Post* clips, hundreds of articles reminding me of how bizarre my job is: the victims and suspects, dangerous slums, prisons and hospitals, twelve-hour shifts spent shivering inside photographers' cars waiting to photograph—or "pop"—celebrities. I had always loved every minute of it. So why was I suddenly so terrible at it?

As I shoved these treasures into the trash bags, I paused on a few headlines, among them the biggest story of my career to date: the time I managed to land an exclusive jailhouse interview with child kidnapper Michael Devlin. The national media were hot on the story, and I was only a senior at Washington University in St. Louis, yet Devlin spoke to me twice. But the story didn't end there. His lawyers went nuts after the article ran, launching a smear campaign against the *Post* and calling for a judicial gag order, while the local and national media began debating my methods on live TV and questioning the ethics of jailhouse interviews and tabloids in general. Paul fielded several tearful phone calls from me during that time, which bound us together, and in the end, both the paper and my editors stood by me. Though the experience had rattled me, it also whetted my appetite, and from then on, I became the resident "jailhouser." Devlin was eventually sentenced to three consecutive lifetimes in prison.

Then there was the butt implant story, "Rear and Present Danger," a headline that still makes me laugh. I had to go undercover as a stripper looking for cheap butt enhancements from a woman who was illegally dispensing them out of a midtown hotel room. As I stood there with my pants around my ankles, I tried not to be insulted when she announced that she would need "a thousand dollars per cheek," twice the amount she charged the woman who had come forward to the *Post*.

Journalism was thrilling; I had always loved living a reality that was more fabulist than fiction, though little did I know that my life was about to become so bizarre as to be worthy of coverage in my own beloved tabloid.

Even though the memory made me smile, I added this clip to the growing trash pile—"where it belongs," I scoffed, despite the fact that those crazy stories had meant the world to me. Though it felt necessary at the moment, this callous throwing away of years' worth of work was completely out of character for me. I was a nostalgic pack rat, who held on to poems that I had written in fourth grade and twenty-some-odd diaries that dated back to junior high. Though there didn't seem to be much of a connection among my bedbug scare, my forgetfulness at work, and my sudden instinct to purge my files, what I didn't know then is that bug obsession can be a sign of psychosis. It's a little-known problem, since those suffering from parasitosis, or Ekbom syndrome, as it's called, are most likely to consult exterminators or dermatologists for their imaginary infestations instead of mental health professionals, and as a result they frequently go undiagnosed. My problem, it turns out, was far vaster than an itchy forearm and a forgotten meeting.

After hours of packing everything away to ensure a bedbug-free zone, I still didn't feel any better. As I knelt by the black garbage bags, I was hit with a terrible ache in the pit of my stomach—that kind of free-floating dread that accompanies heartbreak or death. When I got to my feet, a sharp pain lanced my mind, like a white-hot flash of a migraine, though I had never suffered from one before. As I stumbled to the bathroom, my legs and body just wouldn't react, and I felt as if I were slogging through quicksand. *I must be getting the flu,* I thought.

—◦◦◦—

This might not have been the flu, though, the same way there may have been no bedbugs. But there likely was a pathogen of some sort that had invaded my body, a little germ that set everything in motion. Maybe it came from that businessman who had sneezed on me in the subway a few days before, releasing millions of virus particles onto the rest of us in that subway car? Or maybe it was in something I ate or something that slipped inside me through a tiny wound on my skin, maybe through one of those mysterious bug bites?

There my mind goes again.

The doctors don't actually know how it began for me. What's clear is that if that man had sneezed on you, you'd most likely just get a cold. For me, it flipped my universe upside down and very nearly sent me to an asylum for life.

CHAPTER 2
THE GIRL IN THE BLACK LACE BRA

A few days later, the migraine, the pitch meeting, and the bedbugs all seemed like a distant memory as I awoke, relaxed and content, in my boyfriend's bed. The night before, I had taken Stephen to meet my father and stepmother, Giselle, for the first time, in their magnificent Brooklyn Heights brownstone. It was a big step in our four-month-old relationship. Stephen had met my mom already—my parents had divorced when I was sixteen, and I had always been closer to her, so we saw her more often—but my dad can be intimidating, I know, and he and I had never had a very open relationship. (Though they'd been married for more than a year, Dad and Giselle had only recently told my brother and me about their marriage.) But it had been a warm and pleasant dinner with wine and good food. Stephen and I had left believing that the evening was a success.

Although my dad would later confess that during that first meeting, he had thought of Stephen as more of a placeholder than a long-term boyfriend, I didn't agree at all. We'd only recently begun dating, but Stephen and I had first met six years earlier, when I was eighteen and we worked together at the same record store in Summit, New Jersey. Back then, we passed the workdays with polite banter, but the relationship never went any deeper, mainly because he is seven years my senior (an unthinkable gap for a teenager). Then one night the previous fall, we had run into each other at a mutual friend's party at a bar in the East Village. Clinking our bottles of Sierra Nevada, we bonded over our shared dislike for shorts and our passion for Dylan's *Nashville Skyline*. Stephen was alluring in that languid, stay-out-all-night kind of way: a musician with long, unkempt hair, a skinny smoker's frame, and an encyclopedic knowledge of music. But his eyes, trusting and honest, have always been his most attractive trait. Those eyes, with nothing to hide, made me feel as if I had dated him forever.

That morning, stretched out in his bed in his enormous (by comparison) studio apartment in Jersey City, I realized I had the place to myself. Stephen had already left for band practice and would be gone for the rest of the day, leaving me free to either spend the day there or let myself out. We had exchanged keys about a month earlier. It was the first time I had taken such a step with a boyfriend, but I had no doubt it was right. We felt deeply comfortable together, generally happy, safe, and trusting. As I lay there, however, I was suddenly, unexpectedly, hit with one overpowering thought: *Read his e-mails.*

This irrational jealousy was wholly unlike me; I had never even been tempted to intellectually trespass like this. But without really considering what I was doing, I opened up his MacBook and began to scroll down his inbox. I sorted through months of mundane e-mails until I triumphantly unearthed a recent one from his ex-girlfriend. The subject line was "Do You Like It?" I clicked, my heart pounding furiously in my chest. She had sent him a picture of herself, posing seductively with her lips pursed, showing off a new auburn hairstyle. It didn't look as if Stephen had ever responded. Still, I fought the urge to punch the computer or throw it across the room. Instead of stopping there, though, I indulged my fury and continued digging until I'd dredged up the correspondence that chronicled their yearlong relationship. Most of these e-mails ended with three words: "I love you." Stephen and I hadn't yet said that to each other. I slammed down the laptop screen, enraged, though I couldn't say exactly why. I knew he hadn't talked to her since we started dating, and he had done nothing inappropriate. But now I felt compelled to go look elsewhere for signs of betrayal.

I tiptoed over to his yellow IKEA dresser—and froze. *What if he has cameras going?* Nah. Who secretly videotapes their home while they're away besides overzealous parents spying on new nannies? But the thought persisted: *What if he's watching me? What if this is a test?* Although I was frightened by this foreign paranoia, it didn't stop me from pulling open the drawers and rifling through his clothes, flinging them on the floor, until I found the jackpot: a cardboard box decorated with band stickers and filled with hundreds of letters and pictures, most of them from exes. There was one long framed photo-booth series with his most recent ex-girlfriend: they pouted, looked longingly at each other, laughed, and then kissed. I could see it happening right in front of me, unfolding like a child's flipbook: I was witnessing them falling in love. Next there was a picture of the same girl in a see-through lace bra with her hands on her bony hips. Her hair was bleached blond, but it looked attractive, not whorish. Below that were the letters, a fistful of handwritten notes that went as far back as Stephen's teens. At the top, the same girlfriend gushed about how much she missed him while she was staying in France. She misused the word *their* and spelled *definitely* as *defiantely,* which thrilled me so much that I laughed out loud, a kind of cackle.

Then, as I reached for the next letter, I caught sight of myself in the mirror of the armoire, wearing only a bra and underwear, clutching Stephen's private love letters between my thighs. A stranger stared back from my reflection; my hair was wild and my face distorted and unfamiliar. *I never act like this,* I thought, disgusted. *What is wrong with me? I have never in my life snooped through a boyfriend's things.*

I ran to the bed and opened my cell phone: I had lost two hours. It felt like five minutes. Moments later, the migraine returned, as did the nausea. It was then that I first noticed my left hand felt funny, like an extreme case of pins and needles. I clenched and unclenched my hand, trying to stop the tingling, but it got worse. I raced to the dresser to put away his things so that he wouldn't notice my pilfering, trying to ignore the uncomfortable tingling sensation. Soon though, my left hand went completely numb.

CHAPTER 3
CAROTA

The pins and needles, which persisted unabated over many days, didn't concern me nearly as much as the guilt and bewilderment I felt over my behavior in Stephen's room that Sunday morning. At work the next day, I commissioned the help of the features editor, Mackenzie, a friend who is as prim and put together as a character out of *Mad Men*.

"I did a really bad thing," I confessed to her outside the News Corp. building, huddling under an overhang in an ill-fitting winter coat. "I snooped at Stephen's house. I found all these pictures of his ex-girlfriend. I went through all of his stuff. It was like I was possessed."

She shot me a knowing half-smile, flipping her hair off her shoulders. "That's all? That's really not so bad."

"Mackenzie, it's psycho. Do you think my birth control is causing hormonal changes?" I had recently started using the patch.

"Oh, come on," she countered. "All women, especially New Yorkers, do that, Susannah. We're competitive. Seriously, don't be so hard on yourself. Just try not to do it again." Mackenzie would later admit she was concerned not by the act of snooping itself but by my overreaction to having done it.

I spotted Paul smoking nearby and posed the same question. I could depend on him to tell it to me straight. "No, you're not crazy," he assured me. "And you shouldn't be worried. Every guy keeps pictures or something from their exes. It's the spoils of war," he explained helpfully. Paul could always be counted on for a man's perspective, because he is so singularly male: eats hard (a double cheeseburger with bacon and a side of gravy), gambles hard (he once lost $12,000 on a single hand at the blackjack table at the Borgata in Atlantic City), and parties hard (Johnnie Walker Blue when he's winning, Macallan 12 when he isn't).

When I got to my desk, I noticed that the numbness in my left hand had returned—or maybe it had never left?—and had moved down the left side of my body to my toes. This was perplexing; I couldn't decide if I should be worried, so I called Stephen.

"I can't explain; it just feels numb," I said on the phone, holding my head parallel to my desk because my landline cord was so tangled.

"Is it like pins and needles?" he asked. I heard him strum a few chords on his guitar in the background.

"Maybe? I don't know. It's weird. It's like nothing I've felt before," I said.

"Are you cold?"

"Not particularly."

"Well, if it doesn't go away, you should probably go to a doctor." I rolled my eyes. This coming from the guy who hadn't been to a doctor in years. I needed another opinion. When Stephen and I hung up, I swiveled my chair around to face Angela.

"Did you sneeze or bend over funny?" she asked. Her aunt had recently sneezed and dislocated a disc in her spine, which had caused numbness in her hands.

"I think you should get it checked out," another reporter piped up from her desk nearby. "Maybe I've been watching too many episodes of *Mystery Diagnosis,* but there's a lot of scary shit out there."

I laughed this off at the time, but flickers of doubt danced in my head. Even though my colleagues were professional slingers of hyperbole, hearing the worry in their voices made me start to rethink my laissez-faire attitude. That day during a lunch break, I finally decided to call my gynecologist, Eli Rothstein, who had over time become more of a friend than a medical practitioner; he had even treated my mom when she was pregnant with me.

Most of the time Rothstein was laid back; I was young and generally healthy, so I was accustomed to his telling me everything was normal. But when I described my symptoms, the usual warmth dropped from his voice: "I'd like you to see a neurologist as soon as possible. And I'd like you to stop taking your birth control immediately." He arranged for me to visit a prominent neurologist that afternoon.

Concerned by his reaction, I hailed a cab and headed uptown, the taxi zipping in and out of the early afternoon traffic before dropping me in front of an impressive Upper East Side building where doormen staffed a grand marble lobby. One doorman pointed me to an unmarked wooden door on the right. The contrast between the crystal-chandeliered entrance and the drab office was discomfiting, as if I had jumped back in time to the 1970s. Three unmatched tweed chairs and a light brown flannel couch provided seating. I chose the couch and tried to avoid sinking in at its center. A few paintings hung around the walls of the waiting room: an ink sketch of a godlike man with a long white beard holding an instrument that looked suspiciously like a surgical needle; a pastoral scene; and a court jester. The haphazard decor made me wonder if everything, including the furniture, had been dug up at a garage sale or pilfered from sidewalk castoffs.

Several emphatic signs hung at the receptionist's desk: PLEASE DO NOT USE LOBBY FOR PHONE CALLS OR WAITING FOR PATIENTS!!!!!! ALL COPAYS MUST BE PAID BEFORE SEEING DOCTOR!!!!!!!

"I'm here to see Dr. Bailey," I said. Without a smile and without looking at me, the receptionist shoved a clipboard in my direction. "Fill it out. Wait."

I breezed through the form. Never again would a health history be so simple. Any medications? No. Allergies? No. History of surgery or previous illness? I paused here. About five years ago, I had been diagnosed with melanoma on my lower back. It had been caught early and required only minor surgery to remove. No chemo, nothing else. I jotted this down. Despite this premature cancer scare, I had remained nonchalant, some would say immature, about my health; I was about as far from a hypochondriac as you can get. Usually it took several pleading phone calls from my mom for me to even follow through on my regular doctor's appointments, so it was a big deal that I was here alone and without any prodding. The shock of the gynecologist's uncharacteristic worry had been unnerving. I needed answers.

To keep calm, I fixated on the strangest and most colorful of the paintings—a distorted, abstract human face outlined in black with bright patches of primary colors, red pupils, yellow eyes, blue chin, and a black nose like an arrow. It had a lipless smile and a deranged look in its eyes. This painting would stick in my mind, materializing again several more times in the coming months. Its unsettling, inhuman distortion sometimes soothed me, sometimes antagonized me, sometimes goaded me during my darkest hours. It turned out to be a 1978 Miró titled *Carota,* or carrot in Italian.

"CALLAAHAANN," the nurse brayed, mispronouncing my name. It was a common, excusable mistake. I stepped forward, and she showed me to an empty examination room, then handed me a green cotton gown. After a few moments, a man's baritone voice echoed behind the door: "Knock, knock." Dr. Saul Bailey was a grandfatherly-looking man. He introduced himself, extending his left hand, which was soft but strong. In my own, smaller one it felt meaty, significant. He spoke quickly. "So you're Eli's patient," he began. "Tell me what's going on."

"I don't really know. I have this weird numbness." I waved my left hand at him to illustrate. "And in my foot."

"Hmmm," he said, reading over my chart. "Any history of Lyme disease?"

"Nope." There was something about his demeanor that made me want to reassure him, to say, "Forget it, I'm fine." He somehow made me want not to be a burden.

He nodded. "Okay, then. Let's have a look."

He conducted a typical neurological exam. It would be the first of many hundreds to come. He tested my reflexes with a hammer, constricted my eyes with a light, assessed my muscle strength by pushing his hands against my outstretched arms, and checked my coordination by having me close my eyes and maneuver my fingers to my nose. Eventually he jotted down "normal exam."

"I'd like to draw some blood, do a routine workup, and I'd like you to get an MRI. I'm not seeing anything out of the norm, but just to be safe, I'd like you to get one," he added.

Normally I would have put the MRI off, but today I decided to follow through. A young, lanky lab technician in his early thirties greeted me in the lab's waiting room and walked me toward a changing area. He led me to a private dressing room, offered a cotton gown, and instructed me to take off all my clothes and jewelry, lest they interfere with the machinery. After he left, I disrobed, folded my clothes, removed my lucky gold ring, and dropped it into a lockbox. The ring had been a graduation gift from my stepfather—it was 14K gold with a black hematite cat's eye, which some cultures believe can ward off evil spirits. The tech waited for me outside the changing area, smiling as he guided me to the MRI room, where he helped prop me up on the platform, placed a helmet on my head, tucked a blanket over my bare legs, and then walked out to oversee the procedure from a separate room.

After half an hour of enduring repeated close-range booming inside the machine, I heard the tech's faraway voice: "Good job. We're all set."

The platform moved out of the machine as I pulled off the helmet, removed the blanket, and got to my feet, feeling uncomfortably exposed in just the hospital gown.

The technician grinned at me and leaned his body against the wall. "So what do you do?"

"I'm a reporter for a newspaper," I said.

"Oh yeah, which one?"

"The *New York Post*."

"No way! I've never met a real-life reporter before," he said as we walked back to the changing room. I didn't reply. I put on my clothes as quickly as I could and rushed toward the elevators to avoid another conversation with the tech, who I felt was being awkwardly flirtatious. Unpleasant as they can be, MRIs are largely unremarkable. But something about this visit, especially that innocent exchange with the tech, stayed with me long after the appointment, much like the *Carota* picture. Over time, the tech's mild flirtations teemed with a strange malevolence created entirely by my churning brain.

It wasn't until hours later, when I idly tried to twirl my ring on my still-numb left hand, that I realized the real casualty of that disturbing day. I had left my lucky ring in that lockbox.

—⁓—

"Is it bad that my hand still feels tingly all the time?" I asked Angela again the next day at work. "I just feel numb and not like myself."

"Do you think you have the flu?"

"I feel terrible. I think I have a fever," I said, glancing at my ringless left finger. My nausea matched my anxiety about the ring. I was obsessed by its absence, but I couldn't get up the nerve to call the office and hear that it was gone. Irrationally, I was instead clinging to that empty hope: *Better not to know,* I convinced myself. I also knew I was going to be too sick to make the trek later that night to see Stephen's band, the Morgues, perform at a bar in Greenpoint, Brooklyn, which made me feel worse. Watching me, Angela said, "You don't look too hot. Why don't I walk you home?"

Normally I would have refused her offer, especially because it was Friday evening on deadline, which typically kept us at the office until 10:00 p.m. or later, but I felt so nauseous and sick and mad at myself that I let her escort me. The trip, which should have taken five minutes, today took a half-hour because after practically every other step I had to stop and dry heave. Once we got to my apartment, Angela insisted I phone my doctor to get some answers. "This just isn't normal. You've been sick for too long," she said.

I dialed the after-hours hotline and soon received a phone call back from the gynecologist, Dr. Rothstein.

"I do want to let you know that we've gotten some good news. Yesterday's MRI came back normal. And we've eliminated the possibility that you had a stroke or a blood clot, two things that, frankly, I was worried about because of the birth control."

"That's great."

"Yes, but I want you to stay off the birth control, just to be safe," he said. "The only thing that the MRI showed was a small amount of enlargement of a few lymph nodes in your neck, which leads me to believe that it's some kind of virus. Possibly mononucleosis, though we don't have the blood tests back to prove it yet."

I almost laughed out loud. Mono in my twenties. As I hung up, Angela was looking at me expectantly. "Mono, Angela. Mono."

The tension left her face and she laughed. "Are you kidding me? You have the kissing disease. What are you, like, thirteen?"

CHAPTER 4
THE WRESTLER

Mono. It was a relief to have a word for what plagued me. Though I spent Saturday in bed feeling sorry for myself, I gathered enough strength the next night to join Stephen, his oldest sister, Sheila, and her husband, Roy, at a Ryan Adams show in nearby Montclair. Before the show, we met at a local Irish pub, sitting in the dining area underneath a low-hanging antique chandelier that let off little tufts of light. I ordered fish and chips, though I couldn't even stomach the image of the dish. Stephen, Sheila, and Roy made small talk as I sat there, mute. I had met Sheila and Roy only a few times and hated to imagine what kind of impression I was making, but I couldn't rouse myself to join the conversation. *They must think I have no personality.* When my fish and chips came, I immediately regretted my order. The cod, caked in thick fried batter, seemed to glow. The fat on it glinted in the light from the chandelier. The fries too looked sickeningly greasy. I pushed the food around on my plate, hoping no one would notice I wasn't actually eating anything.

We arrived early for the show, but the music hall was already crowded. Stephen wanted to be as close to the stage as possible, so he pushed forward through the crowd. I tried following him, but as I moved deeper into the horde of thirtysomething men, I grew dizzy and queasy.

I called out to him, "I can't do this!"

Stephen gave up his mission and joined me at the back of the floor by a pillar, which I needed to support my weight. My purse felt as if it weighed forty pounds, and I struggled to balance it on my shoulder because there wasn't enough space around me to lay it on the floor.

The background music swelled. I love Ryan Adams and tried to cheer but could only clap my hands weakly. Two five-foot-tall neon blue roses hung in the background behind the band, burning into my vision. I felt the pulse of the crowd. A man to my left lit up a joint, and the sweet smell of smoke made me gag. The breath of the man and woman behind me flared hotly on my neck. I couldn't focus on the music. The show was torture.

Afterward we piled into Sheila's car so she could drive us back to Stephen's apartment in Jersey City. The three of them talked about how incredible the band had been, but I stayed silent. My shyness struck Stephen as strange; I was never one to keep my opinions to myself.

"Did you like the show?" Stephen nudged, reaching out for my hand.

"I can't really remember it."

After that weekend, I took three more consecutive days off work. That was a lot for anyone, but especially for a newbie reporter. Even when the *Post* kept me out past 4:00 a.m. working on Meatpacking District club stories, I always made it to the office right on time a few hours later. I never took sick days.

I decided to finally share my diagnosis with my mother, who was distressed when I told her about the numbness, particularly because it was only on one side of the body. I assured her it was only because of the mono. My father seemed less concerned on the phone, but on my third day off he insisted on coming into Manhattan to see me. We met at an empty AMC Theater in Times Square for an early showing of *The Wrestler*.

"I used to try to forget about you," Randy "the Ram," a washed-up pro wrestler played by a haggard Mickey Rourke, says to his daughter. "I used to try to pretend that you didn't exist, but I can't. You're my little girl. And now I'm an old broken-down piece of meat and I'm alone. And I deserve to be all alone. I just don't want you to hate me." Hot, wet tears ran down my cheeks.

Embarrassed, I tried to control the heaving in my chest, but the exertion made me feel worse. Without saying a word to my father, I ran from my seat to the theater's bathroom, where I hid in a locked stall and allowed myself to weep until the feeling passed. After a moment, I collected myself and headed out to wash my hands and face, ignoring the concerned rubbernecking of the middle-aged blond at a nearby sink. When she left, I stared at my image in the mirror. Was Mickey Rourke really getting to me? Or was it the whole father-daughter thing? My dad was far from affectionate, habitually avoiding using words like "I love you," even with his children. It was a learned deficiency. The one time he had kissed his own father was when my grandfather was on his deathbed. And now he was taking time out of his busy schedule to sit beside me in an empty theater. So, yeah, it was unsettling.

Get yourself together, I mouthed. *You're acting ridiculous.*

I rejoined my father, who didn't seem to have noticed my emotional outburst, and sat through the remaining portion of the movie without another breakdown. After the closing credits, my father insisted on walking me to my apartment, offering to check it out because of the bedbug scare, though it was clear he was mainly concerned about my health and wanted to spend more time with me.

"So *they* say you have mono, huh?" he asked. Unlike my mother, who reviewed *New York* magazine's list of best doctors religiously, my father had always distrusted medical authority. I nodded and shrugged my shoulders.

When we got near my apartment, however, my stomach filled with that inexplicable but now-familiar dread. I suddenly realized that I didn't want him to come inside. Like most fathers, he had chastised me when I was a teenager about allowing my room to get filthy, so I was used to that. But today I felt ashamed, as if the room was a metaphor for my screwed-up life. I dreaded the idea of his seeing how I was living.

"What the hell is that smell?" he said as I unlocked the door.

Shit. I grabbed a plastic Duane Reade bag by the door. "I forgot to throw out the kitty litter."

"Susannah. You've got to get yourself together. You can't live like this. You're an adult."

We both stood in the doorway, looking at my studio. He was right: it was squalid. Dirty clothes littered the floor. The trash can was overflowing. And the black garbage bags, which I'd packed during the bedbug scare and before the exterminator had come to spray three weeks earlier, still covered the room. No bedbugs were found, and no more bites had surfaced. By now I was convinced it was over—and a small part of me had begun to wonder if they had ever been there at all.

CHAPTER 5
COLD ROSES

I returned to work the next day, a Thursday, which gave me just enough time to finish up a story and pitch two more. Neither passed muster.

"Please do LexisNexis searches first," Steve wrote, responding to my new pitches.

Insecurity is part of the job, I told myself. Reporters exist in a state of constant self-doubt: sometimes we have disastrous weeks when stories don't pan out or sources clam up; other times we have killer ones, when even the seemingly impossible works out in our favor. There are times when you feel like the best in the business, and other times when you're certain that you're a complete and total hack and should start looking for an office job. But in the end, the ups and downs even out. So why was everything in such upheaval for me? It had been weeks since I felt comfortable in my own journalist skin, and that frightened me.

Frustrated by my sloppy performance, I asked to go home early, again, hoping it was just the mono. Maybe a good night's sleep would finally get me back to my usual self.

That night I tossed and turned, filled with misgivings about my life. When my alarm clock rang the next morning, I hit the snooze button and decided to call in sick again. After a few more hours of sleep, I woke up rested and calm, as if the whole mono thing had been a distant nightmare. The weekend now loomed brightly on the horizon. I phoned Stephen.

"Let's go to Vermont." It was a statement, not a question. Weeks earlier we had had plans to go to Vermont and stay at my stepbrother's house, but since I had gotten sick, the trip had been postponed indefinitely. Sensing that I still wasn't my old self, Stephen was offering reasons that we shouldn't rush into the trip when a blocked call beeped in on the other line. It was Dr. Rothstein.

"The blood test results came back. You are not positive for mononucleosis," he said. "How are you feeling?"

"So much better."

"Okay, then, it must have been some garden-variety virus that's now out of your system."

Invigorated, I called Stephen back, insisting that we pack our bags and go away for the weekend. He caved. That afternoon we borrowed my mom's black Subaru and drove four hours north to Arlington, Vermont. It was a perfect weekend: Saturday and Sunday mornings we went to a quaint local restaurant called Up For Breakfast, shopped at outlet malls, and hit the slopes—or, rather, Stephen snowboarded as I read *Great Expectations* in the lodge. On Sunday a snowstorm hit, so we were happily forced to stay another day, which meant more time off from work. Finally I agreed to ski, and Stephen led me to the top of a small mountain.

I had skied a few times before and never found the intermediate slopes difficult to manage, though I was hardly an expert. But this time, as the wind whipped my face and the snowflakes burned my cheeks, the mountain suddenly seemed far steeper than ever before. It loomed out below me, long, narrow, and threatening. I felt instantly helpless, and I panicked, a kind of deep-seated fight-or-flight fear that I had read about but never experienced.

"Ready?" Stephen's voice sounded distant in the howling winds. My heart pounded in my ears, as I raced through ever-more-terrible scenarios: *What if I never make it down? What if Stephen leaves me here? What if they never find my body?*

"I can't do this," I shouted. "I don't want to. Please don't make me do this."

"Come on!" he said, but stopped his cajoling when he sensed my anxiety. "It's okay. I promise you'll be okay. We'll take it slow."

I headed nervously down the mountain with Stephen following. Midway down, I picked up speed, feeling silly about my terror from moments before. Safe at the bottom a few minutes later, though, I recognized that this panic had been far more critical than just a fear of heights. Still, I said nothing further about it to Stephen.

Monday night, back at my mother's house in New Jersey, I was still having trouble sleeping, but now instead of nervous, I felt nostalgic. I riffled through old clothes and discovered I finally fit into pants that I'd only been able to pull up to my midthigh since sophomore year in high school. *I must be doing something right,* I thought gleefully.

I would soon learn firsthand that this kind of illness often ebbs and flows, leaving the sufferer convinced that the worst is over, even when it's only retreating for a moment before pouncing again.

CHAPTER 6

AMERICA'S MOST WANTED

The next Tuesday morning at work, my office phone rang. It was Steve. He seemed to have forgiven me for my recent absence and displays of ineptitude, or at least had decided to give me another shot: "I want you to interview John Walsh tomorrow morning when he comes in for a Fox News interview. He's working on a new episode about drug-smuggling submarines that I think could be a fun page lead."

"Sure," I said, trying to muster up the enthusiasm that had once come so naturally. It did sound exciting to interview the host of *America's Most Wanted,* but I couldn't seem to focus. The first thing I needed to do was a clip search, so I called the *Post*'s librarian, Liz. She is a researcher by day, Wiccan priestess by night. Inexplicably, instead of asking for a search, I requested a tarot reading.

"Come on by," she said languidly.

Liz practiced modern witchcraft using candles, spells, and potions. She had recently been appointed Third Degree High Priestess, meaning she was able to teach the craft. She wore rows of pentacles and flowing Stevie Nicks–style clothes, and even donned a black cape in winter. She smelled of incense and patchouli and had drooping, trustworthy, puppy eyes. There was something attractive about her energy, and despite my innate skepticism of witchcraft and religion overall, I found myself wanting to believe.

"I need your help," I said. "Things are not going well. Will you do a reading?"

"Hmmm," she said, laying out a deck of tarot cards. "Hmmm." She drew out each syllable. "So I see good things. Positive stuff.

You're going to have some sort of a job change. Something free-lance outside the *Post*. Financially, I see good things for you."

Waves of calm coursed through my system as I concentrated on her words. I had needed someone to tell me that I was going to be okay, that these odd setbacks were just blips on the radar of my life. In retrospect, Liz may not have been the right person to go to for this kind of reassurance.

"Oh, man. I feel all floaty," Liz added.

"Yeah, me too." I did.

When I returned to my desk, Angela looked depressed. A fellow *Post* reporter, our resident renaissance man who covered all sorts of beats for the paper, had passed away from melanoma. An e-mail was circulating throughout the newsroom, outlining the funeral arrangements for that Friday. He had been only fifty-three years old. It made me think of my own melanoma diagnosis, and for the rest of the day, even as I should have been researching John Walsh, I couldn't force the sad news out of my mind.

The next morning, after another sleepless night, I used the few remaining moments I had to prepare for the interview to Google melanoma relapse rates instead. I was completely unprepared when 9:50 a.m. hit, but I headed out to meet Walsh in an empty office down the hall anyway, hoping I could just wing it. As I walked through the hallway, framed *Post* front pages began to close in on me, their headlines contracting and expanding.

BILL CHEATED ON ME!

SPACESHIP EXPLODES MIDAIR, ALL 7 DIE

DIANA DEAD

THE KINK AND I

CHILLARY

The pages were breathing visibly, inhaling and exhaling all around me. My perspective had narrowed, as if I were looking down the hallway through a viewfinder. The fluorescent lights flickered, and the walls tightened claustrophobically around me. As the walls caved in, the ceiling stretched sky-high until I felt as if I were in a cathedral. I put my hand to my chest to quell my racing heart and told myself to breathe. I wasn't frightened; it felt more like the sterile rush of looking down from the window of a hundred-story skyscraper, knowing you won't fall.

Finally I reached the office where Walsh was waiting for me. He still had the makeup on from his Fox News interview, and it had melted a bit under the bright lights of the studio.

"Hi, John, my name is Susannah Cahalan. I'm the *Post* reporter."

As soon as I saw him, I started wondering, oddly, if Walsh was thinking right then about his murdered son, Adam, who had been abducted from a department store in 1981 and found decapitated later that year. My mind wandered through this macabre subject as I stood smiling blandly at him and his manicured publicist.

"Hello," the publicist said, breaking my train of thought.

"Oh, hi! Yes. My name is Susannah Cahalan. I'm the reporter. The reporter on the story. You know, on the drug smuggling, drug smuggling—"

Walsh interrupted here. "Submarines, yes."

"He only has five minutes, so we should probably get going," the publicist said, a hint of annoyance evident in her tone.

"Many South American drug smugglers are making home-made submarines," Walsh began. "Well, actually, they aren't in fact submarines but submersible crafts that look like submarines." I jotted notes: "Columbian" [sic], "homemade," "track about ten a . . ." "Drug boats, we must stop boats . . ." I couldn't follow what he was saying, so I mainly jotted down disassociated words to make it seem as if I was paying attention.

"It is very cunning."

I laughed uproariously at this line, though I didn't know then and still can't figure out what about that word seemed so funny. The publicist shot me a puzzled look before announcing, "I'm sorry, I have to interrupt the interview. John needs to go."

"I'll walk you out," I said with pressured enthusiasm and led them to the elevators. But as I walked, I could barely maintain my balance, bumping into the walls of the hallway, reaching for the door to open it for them but missing the handle by a solid foot.

"Thank you, thank you. I'm a huge fan, huge fan. HUGE fan," I gushed, as we waited at the elevators.

Walsh smiled with kindness, possibly accustomed to this type of eccentric effusiveness that was in fact divorced from my typical interview style.

"It was a pleasure," he said.

I still don't know—and probably never will—what he really thought of the strange *Post* reporter, especially because the story never ran. This would be the last interview I conducted for seven months.

CHAPTER 7

ON THE ROAD AGAIN

I don't remember how I got home after the interview or how I filled the hours in the wake of yet another professional debacle, but after still another sleepless night—it had now been over a week since I'd slept fully—I headed to the office. It was a gorgeous early March morning, the sun was out, and the temperature was a crisp thirty degrees. I had walked through Times Square twice a day for six months, but today, once I hit the rows of billboards at its center I was accosted by its garish colors. I tried to look away, to shield myself from shock waves of pigment, but I couldn't. The bright blue wedge of an Eclipse gum sign emitted electric swirls of aqua and made the hair on the back of my neck stand up. I could feel the colors vibrating in my toes. There seemed to be something exquisite about that rush; it was simultaneously enervating and thrilling. But the thrill lasted only a moment when, to my left, the moving scroll of "Welcomes you to Times Square" caught my attention and made me want to retch in the middle of the street. M&M's on an animated billboard to my left pirouetted before me, forging a massive migraine in my temples. Helpless in the face of this onslaught, I covered my eyes with mittenless hands, stumbling up Forty-Eighth Street as if I had just gotten off a death-defying roller coaster, until I hit the newsroom, where the lights still felt bright but less aggressive.

"Angela, I have to tell you something strange," I whispered, concerned that people might be listening in, thinking I was crazy. "I see bright colors. The colors hurt my eyes."

"What do you mean?" she asked, worry evident in her smile. Every day my behavior had been growing increasingly erratic.

But it wasn't until this morning that my ramblings had begun to frighten her.

"Times Square. The colors, the billboards: they're so bright. Brighter than I've ever seen them before."

"You must be really hung over." She laughed nervously.

"I didn't drink. I think I'm losing my mind."

"If you're really concerned, I think you should go back and see a doctor."

There's something wrong with me. This is how a crazy person acts.

Frustrated with my inability to communicate what was happening to me, I slammed my hands down on the keyboard. The computer glowed back at me, bright and angry. I looked at Angela to see if she saw it too, but she was busy with her e-mail.

"I can't do this!" I shouted.

"Susannah, Susannah. Hey, what's going on?" Angela asked, surprised by the outburst. I had never been histrionic, and now that everyone was staring at me, I felt humiliated and on display, and hot tears streamed down my face and onto my blouse. "Why are you crying?"

I shrugged off the question, too embarrassed to go into details I didn't understand.

"Do you want to go out for a walk or something? Grab a coffee?"

"No, no. I don't know what's wrong with me. I'm all fucked up. I'm crying for no reason," I sobbed. As the crying spell took over my whole body, I became prisoner to it. The more I told myself to stop, the more powerful the sensation became. What was causing these hysterics? I fixated on anything my mind could grasp, picking apart the minutiae of my life, anything that felt uncertain. *I'm bad at my job. Stephen doesn't love me. I'm broke. I'm crazy. I'm stupid.* Many of my colleagues were now returning to the office, dressed in black from the reporter's funeral, which I had not attended because I was too consumed by my own problems. *Was this the reason I was crying? I hardly knew the man. Was I crying for myself? Over the possibility that I might be next?*

Another reporter, who sat directly across from Angela, turned around. "Susannah, are you okay?"

I hated the attention. I shot her a derisive look, heavy with loathing. "Stop. It."

The tears continued down my face, but I was surprised to realize that instantly I was no longer sad. I was fine. Not fine. Happy. No, not happy, sublime, better than I had ever felt in my entire life. The tears kept coming, but now I was laughing. A pulse of warmth shot up my spine. I wanted to dance or sing, something, anything except sit here and wallow in imaginary misery. I ran to the bathroom to splash some water on my face. As the cold water flowed, the bathroom stalls suddenly looked alien to me. How was it that civilization had gotten so far but we still defecated in such close proximity to one another? I looked at the stalls and, hearing the flushing of toilets, I could not believe that I had ever used one before.

When I got back to my desk, my emotions now relatively stable, I called Mackenzie, who had been so helpful with my snooping problem weeks ago, and asked her to meet me downstairs. I wanted her opinion on what had just happened to me. When I found her behind the News Corp. building, I noticed that she too was wearing black and had just arrived from the reporter's funeral. I suddenly felt ashamed for being so self-obsessed.

"I'm so sorry to bother you when you're suffering," I said. "I know it's really selfish of me to behave like this right now."

"Don't worry about it. What's going on?" she asked.

"I just. I just. Do you ever not feel like yourself?"

She laughed. "I hardly ever feel like myself."

"But this is different. Something is really wrong. I'm seeing bright colors, crying uncontrollably. I can't control myself," I repeated, wiping away the remaining moisture from my swollen eyes. "Do you think I'm having a nervous breakdown? Do you think I'm going nuts?"

"Look, Susannah, this isn't something you can do yourself. You really need to just go see a doctor. I think you should write down all your symptoms, as if you were going to write up a story about it. Don't leave anything out. As you know, even the smallest details can turn out to be the most important."

It was genius. I nearly ran away from her to go upstairs and start writing. But when I got to my desk, I wrote only the following:

Insomnia
_____
Vision

Then I began doodling, though I don't remember scrawling out the drawing or what prompted it:

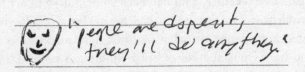

"People are desperate, they'll do anything," I'd written. Abruptly I stopped writing and began to clear everything off my desk—all the water bottles, the half-empty coffee cups, and the old articles that I would never read again. I lugged armfuls of books that I'd been saving for reasons I could no longer remember to the floor's Dumpster and discarded them all, as if they were evidence that I was a hoarder who had been unraveling for months. I suddenly felt in control of every part of my life. That buoyant happiness had returned. But even then I recognized it was a perilous happiness. I feared that if I didn't express it and appreciate it, the emotion would blaze and burn away as quickly as it came.

When I got back to my desk, I slammed my hands down on top of it.

"Everything is going to be great!" I announced, ignoring Angela's astonishment. I sauntered over to Paul's desk, high on my brand-new, wonderfully simple theory on life.

"Let's go downstairs for a smoke!"

As we took the elevator, Paul said, "You look much better."

"Thanks, Paul. I feel so much better. I feel like myself again, and I have so much to talk to you about." We lit cigarettes. "You know, it's finally dawned on me what is wrong. I want to do more stories. Better stories. Bigger stories. Not the feature bullshit. The real stuff. The real hard-hitting investigations."

"Well, that's great," Paul said, but he also looked concerned. "Are you okay? You're talking a mile a minute."

"Sorry. I'm just so excited!"

"I'm glad to hear you're excited, you know, because some people had told me that you've been upset at your desk and you've been so sick the past month."

"That's over. I've seriously figured it out."

"Hey, have you talked to your mom recently?" Paul asked.

"Yeah, a few days ago. Why?"

"Just curious."

Paul was busy building a mental picture, ready to relate to Angela what he felt were the beginning signs of a breakdown. He had once seen another reporter whom he cared about fall apart. She began wearing bright, inappropriate makeup and acting strange, and she was later diagnosed with schizophrenia.

After ten minutes of my ramblings, Paul headed back inside and called Angela. "Someone needs to call her mom or someone. This just isn't right."

While Paul was upstairs talking to Angela, I stayed outside. If anyone looked at me then, they would have assumed that I was deep in thought or working out a story in my head—nothing out of the ordinary. But in fact I was far away. The pendulum had swung again, and now I felt wobbly and height-sick, that same feeling I'd had at the top of the mountain in Vermont, except without the terror. I floated above the crowd of News Corp. employees. I saw the top of my own head, so close that I could almost reach out and touch myself. I saw Liz, the Wiccan librarian, and felt my "self" reenter my grounded body.

"Liz, Liz!" I shouted. "I need to talk to you!"

She stopped. "Oh, hey, Susannah. How's it going?"

There was no time for pleasantries. "Liz, did you ever feel like you're here but you're not here?"

"Sure, all the time," she said.

"No, no, you don't understand. I can see myself from above, like I'm floating above myself looking down," I said, wringing my hands.

"That's normal," she said.

"No, no. Like you're outside of yourself looking in."

"Sure, sure."

"Like you're in your own world. Like you're not in this world."

"I know what you're saying. It's probably just residue from the astral travel you experienced during the reading we did yesterday. I think I may have taken you to another realm. I apologize for that. Just try to relax and embrace it."

Meanwhile, Angela, worried about my erratic behavior, got permission from Paul to take me to the bar at a nearby Marriott hotel for a drink—and to tease some more information out of me about why I was acting so out of character. When I returned to the newsroom, Angela convinced me to gather my things and join her on a walk a few blocks north up Times Square to the hotel bar. We walked into the hotel's main entranceway through revolving doors and stood beside a group of tourists waiting to take the transparent elevators to the eighth-floor bar, but the crowd bothered me. There were too many people around. I couldn't breathe.

"Can we please take the escalator?" I begged Angela.

"Of course."

The escalators, decorated on each side with dozens of glowing bulbs, only intensified my jitters. I tried to ignore the heart palpitations and the sweat forming on my brow. Angela stood a few steps above, looking concerned. I could feel the pressure of fear rise in my chest, and suddenly I was crying again.

At the third floor, I had to get off the escalator to compose myself because I was sobbing so hard. Angela put her arm on my shoulder. In total, I had to get off the escalator three times to steady myself from sobbing during that eight-floor trip.

Finally we reached the bar floor. The rugs, which looked as if they belonged in an avant-garde production of *Lawrence of Arabia,* swirled before me. The harder I stared, the more the abstract patterns merged. I tried to ignore it. The hundred-plus-seat bar, which looked down over Times Square, was almost completely empty, with only a few groups of businessmen dotting the chairs around the entranceway. When we walked in, I was still bawling, and one group looked up from their cocktails and gawked at me, which made me feel worse and more pathetic. The tears kept coming, though I had no clue why. We positioned ourselves in the center of the room at seats with high chairs, far away from the other patrons. I didn't know what I wanted, so Angela ordered a sauvignon blanc for me and an Anchor Steam for herself.

"So what's really going on?" she asked, taking a small sip of her amber-colored beer.

"So many things. The job. I'm terrible at it. Stephen, he doesn't love me. Everything is falling apart. Nothing makes sense," I said, holding the wineglass like a comforting habit but not drinking.

"I understand. You're young. You have this stressful job and a new boyfriend. It's all up in the air. That's scary. But is it really enough to make you feel this upset?"

She was right. I had been thinking about all of that, but it was a struggle to make one detail fit well enough to solve the entire problem, like jamming together pieces from incongruent sets of puzzles. "There's something else," I agreed. "But I don't know what it is."

~~~

When I got home at seven that night, Stephen was already waiting for me. Instead of telling him I'd been out with Angela, I lied and told him I had been at work, convinced that I needed to hide my perplexing behavior from him, even though Angela had urged me to just tell him the truth. But I did warn him that I wasn't acting like myself and hadn't been sleeping well.

"Don't worry," he responded. "I'll open a bottle of wine. That will put you to sleep."

I felt guilty as I watched Stephen methodically stir the sauce for shrimp fra diavolo with a kitchen towel tucked in his pant loops. Stephen was a naturally skilled and inventive cook, but I couldn't enjoy the pampering tonight; instead, I stood up and paced. My thoughts were running wild from guilt to love to repulsion and then back again. I couldn't keep them straight, so I moved my body to quiet my mind. Most of all, I didn't want him to see me in this state.

"You know, I haven't really slept in a while," I announced. In fact, I couldn't remember the last time I had slept. I had gone without real sleep for at least three days, and the insomnia had been plaguing me for weeks, on and off. "I might make it hard for you to sleep."

He looked up from the pasta and smiled. "Don't worry. You'll sleep better with me around."

He handed me a plate with pasta and a healthy helping of parmesan. My stomach turned at the sight, and when I tasted the shrimp, I almost gagged. I pushed the pasta around on my plate as he devoured his. I watched him, trying to hide my disgust.

"What? You don't like it?" he asked, hurt.

"No, it's not that. I'm just not hungry. Great leftovers," I said cheerfully, while having to physically restrain myself from pacing around the apartment. I couldn't stay with one thought; my mind was flooded with different desires, but especially the urge to escape. Eventually I relaxed enough to lie down on my couch bed with Stephen. He poured me a glass of wine, but I left it on the windowsill. Maybe I knew on some primal level that it would have been bad for my state of mind. Instead, I chain-smoked cigarettes, one after another, down to their nubs.

"You're a smoking fiend tonight," he said, putting his own cigarette out. "Maybe that's why you're not hungry."

"Yeah, I should stop," I said. "I feel like my heart is beating out of my chest."

I handed Stephen the remote, and he flipped the channel to PBS. As his heavy breathing turned into all-out snores, *Spain . . . on the Road Again* came on, the reality show that followed actress Gwyneth Paltrow, chef Mario Batali, and *New York Times* food critic Mark Bittman through Spain. *God, not Gwyneth Paltrow,* I thought, but was too lazy to change the channel. As Batali ate luscious eggs and meat, she toyed with a thin goat's-milk yogurt, and when he offered her a bite of his dish, she demurred.

"That's nice to have at seven in the morning," she said sarcastically. You could just tell how disgusted she was by his belly.

As I watched her nibble on her yogurt, my stomach turned. I thought about how little I had eaten in the past week.

"Hold on," he retorted. "I can't see you on that high horse of yours."

I laughed right before everything went hazy.

Gwyneth Paltrow.

Eggs and meat.

Darkness.

CHAPTER 8
OUT-OF-BODY EXPERIENCE

As Stephen later described that nightmarish scene, I had woken him up with a strange series of low moans, resonating among the sounds from the TV. At first he thought I was grinding my teeth, but when the grinding noises became a high-pitched squeak, like sandpaper rubbed against metal, and then turned into deep, *Sling Blade*-like grunts, he knew something was wrong. He thought maybe I was having trouble sleeping, but when he turned over to face me, I was sitting upright, my eyes wide open, dilated but unseeing.

"Hey, what's wrong?"

No response.

When he suggested I try to relax, I turned to face him, staring past him like I was possessed. My arms suddenly whipped straight out in front of me, like a mummy, as my eyes rolled back and my body stiffened. I was gasping for air. My body continued to stiffen as I inhaled repeatedly, with no exhale. Blood and foam began to spurt out of my mouth through clenched teeth. Terrified, Stephen stifled a panicked cry and for a second he stared, frozen, at my shaking body.

Finally, he jumped into action—though he'd never seen a seizure before, he knew what to do. He laid me down, moving my head to the side so that I wouldn't choke, and raced for his phone to dial 911.

I would never regain any memories of this seizure, or the ones to come. This moment, my first serious blackout, marked the line between sanity and insanity. Though I would have moments of lucidity over the coming weeks, I would never again be the same person. This was the start of the dark period of my illness, as I began an existence in purgatory between the real world and a cloudy, fictitious realm made up of hallucinations and paranoia. From this point on, I would increasingly be forced to rely on outside sources to piece together this "lost time."

As I later learned, this seizure was merely the most dramatic and recognizable of a series of seizures I'd been experiencing for days already. Everything that had been happening to me in recent weeks was part of a larger, fiercer battle taking place at the most basic level inside my brain.

The healthy brain is a symphony of 100 billion neurons, the actions of each individual brain cell harmonizing into a whole that enables thoughts, movements, memories, or even just a sneeze. But it takes only one dissonant instrument to mar the cohesion of a symphony. When neurons begin to play nonstop, out of tune, and all at once because of disease, trauma, tumor, lack of sleep, or even alcohol withdrawal, the cacophonous result can be a seizure.

For some people, the result is a "tonic-clonic" seizure like the one Stephen witnessed, characterized by loss of consciousness or muscle rigidity and a strange, often synchronized dance of involuntary movements—my terrifying zombie moves. Others may have more subtle seizures, which are characterized by staring episodes, foggy consciousness, and repetitive mouth or body movements. The long-term ramifications of untreated seizures can include cognitive defects and even death.

The type and severity of a seizure depend on where the neural dysfunction is focused in the brain: if it is in the visual cortex, the person experiences optical distortions, such as visual hallucinations; if it is in the motor areas of the frontal cortex, the person exhibits strange, zombie-like movements; and so forth.

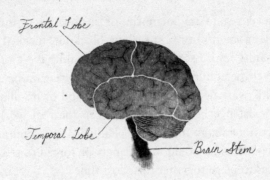

Frontal Lobe

Temporal Lobe

Brain Stem

Along with the violent tonic-clonic seizure, it turned out I had also been experiencing complex partial seizures because of overstimulation in my temporal lobes, generally considered to be the most "ticklish" part of the brain. The temporal lobe houses the ancient structures of the hippocampus and the amygdala, the parts of the brain responsible for emotion and memory. The symptoms from this type of seizure can range from a "Christmas morning" feeling of euphoria to sexual arousal to religious experiences. Often people report feeling déjà vu and its opposite, something called jamais vu, when everything seems unfamiliar, such as my feeling of alienation in the office bathroom; seeing halos of light or viewing the world as if it is bizarrely out of proportion (known as the Alice in Wonderland effect), which is what was happening while I was on my way to interview John Walsh; and experiencing photophobia, an extreme sensitivity to light, like my visions in Times Square. These are all common symptoms or precedents of temporal lobe seizures.

A small subset of those with temporal lobe epilepsy—about 5 to 6 percent—report an out-of-body experience, a feeling described as being removed from your body and able to look at yourself, usually from above.

There I am on a gurney.

There I am being loaded into the ambulance as Stephen holds my hands.

There I am entering a hospital.

Here I am. Floating above the scene, looking down. I am calm. There is no fear.

CHAPTER 9

A TOUCH OF MADNESS

When I gained consciousness the first thing I saw was a homeless man vomiting just a few feet away in a brightly lit hospital room. In one corner, another man, bloodied, beaten, and handcuffed to the bed, was flanked by two police officers.

Am I dead? Anger at my surroundings welled up inside me. *How dare they put me here.* I was too incensed to be terrified, and so I lashed out. I hadn't felt like myself for weeks, but the real damage to my personality was only now bubbling to the surface. Looking back at this time, I see that I'd begun to surrender to the disease, allowing all the aspects of my personality that I value—patience, kindness, and courteousness—to evaporate. I was a slave to the machinations of my aberrant brain. We are, in the end, a sum of our parts, and when the body fails, all the virtues we hold dear go with it.

I am not dead yet. I am dying because of him, because of that lab technician. I convinced myself that the tech who may have flirted with me when I had my MRI was clearly behind all this.

"Get me out of this room NOW," I commanded. Stephen held my hand, looking frightened by the imperiousness in my voice. "I will NOT stay in this room."

I will not die here. I will not die with these freaks.

A doctor approached my bedside. "Yes, we will move you right away." I was triumphant, delighted by my newfound power. *People listen when I speak.* Instead of worrying that my life was out of control, I began to focus on anything that made me feel strong. A nurse and a male assistant wheeled my bed out of the room and into a nearby private one. As the bed moved, I clutched Stephen's hand. I felt so sorry for him. He didn't know that I was dying.

"I don't want you to get upset," I said softly. "But I'm dying of melanoma."

Stephen looked spent. "Stop it, Susannah. Don't say that. You don't know what's wrong." I noticed tears welling up in his eyes. *He can't handle it.* Suddenly the outrage returned.

"I do know what's wrong!" I yelled. "I'm going to sue him! I'm going to take him for all he's worth. He thinks he can hit on me and just let me die? He can't just do that. No, I'm going to destroy him in court!"

Stephen withdrew his hand swiftly, as if he'd been burned. "Susannah, please stay calm. I don't know what you're talking about."

"The MRI guy! He hit on me! He didn't catch the melanoma. I'm suing!"

The young resident interrupted me mid-rant. "This is something you might want to look into when you get home. If you need a good dermatologist, I would be happy to recommend one. Unfortunately, there's nothing more we can do here." The hospital had already conducted a CT scan, a basic neurological exam, and a blood test. "We have to discharge you and advise that you see a neurologist first thing tomorrow."

"Discharged?" Stephen interjected. "You're letting her go? But you don't know what's wrong, and it could happen again. How can you just let her go?"

"I'm sorry, but seizures are fairly common. Sometimes they just happen and never happen again. But this is an emergency room, and we can't just keep her to see. I'm sorry. My advice is to see a neurologist first thing tomorrow morning."

"I'm still suing that guy!"

The doctor nodded patiently and departed to address the gunshot wounds and drug overdoses that awaited him.

"I have to call your mom," Stephen said.

"You don't have to do that," I insisted, my voice mellowing as I returned, almost instantly, to my old self. Manic episodes can fade away as quickly as they arise. "I don't want her to worry." Mom was a worrier by nature, and I had tried to spare her the full story of what was happening to me so far.

"I have to," he insisted and coaxed her home number out of me. He stepped into the hallway and waited two interminably long rings before Allen, my stepfather, picked up the phone.

"Hello," he said groggily in his thick Bronx accent.

"Allen, it's Stephen. I'm at the hospital. Susannah had a seizure, but she's doing fine."

In the background, my mom shouted, "Allen, what is it?"

"She's going to be okay. They're discharging her," Stephen continued.

Despite my mom's rising panic, Allen maintained his composure, telling Stephen to go back home and sleep. They would come in the morning. When he hung up the phone, my mom and Allen looked at each other. It was Friday the Thirteenth.

My mom felt the foreboding, and she began to cry uncontrollably, certain that something was seriously wrong. It was the first and last time she would allow herself to completely succumb to her emotions in the frightening months that followed.

First thing the next morning, while Allen scouted the street for parking, my mom arrived at my apartment door looking sharp, as always. Her frenetic energy, however, was palpable. She was terrified of even hearing about cancer on the radio, and now she had to cope with her own daughter's mysterious seizure. I watched from the bed as she wrung her beautifully shaped hands, the feature I most adored about her, lobbing question after question at Stephen about the night in the hospital.

"Did they give any explanation? What kind of doctor saw her? Did they do an MRI?"

Allen came around behind her and massaged her earlobe, a habit of his to calm people he loves. She unwound the instant he touched her. Allen is her third husband, after my dad: her first husband was an architect, and the marriage didn't work for a number of reasons, in part because my mom, very much a feminist of the 1970s, didn't want children. She wanted to focus instead on her career at Manhattan's district attorney's office, where she still worked. When she met my father, she left her first husband and together they had my brother, James, and me. Despite having had kids together, their relationship was ill fated from the start. Both were as hot-tempered as they were stubborn, yet they managed to make their marriage last nearly two decades before they divorced.

My mom and Allen had met thirty years ago at the district attorney's office, long before she married my dad. Allen had won her over as a friend with his loyalty and devotion. He eventually became her key confidant in and out of the DA's office and through her divorce with my father. Allen's brother was schizophrenic, and as a result Allen had turned inward, maintaining only a few important friendships and living primarily in his own world. He was animated with his closest loved ones, gesticulating wildly with his hands and laughing a contagious guffaw; with outsiders, he could be quiet and aloof, to the point of seeming rude. But his warmth and calm, not to mention his experience with mental illness, would prove invaluable over the coming weeks.

Before my seizure, he and my mom had developed a theory culled from the few things that they knew about my month of strange behavior. They suspected I was having a nervous breakdown, prompted by stress at work and the responsibilities of living on my own. The seizure didn't fit into that scenario, though, and now they were even more concerned. After some debate, they decided it would be safest for me to come home with them to Summit, New Jersey, where they could look after me.

Stephen, my mom, and Allen used various tactics to try to get me out of bed, but I refused to budge. To me, the most important thing was to stay in my own apartment, no matter what: going back to my parents' house would make me feel like a child. As badly as I needed it, help was the last thing I wanted. Somehow, though, their combined forces managed to get me out of my house and into the Subaru.

. . .

Summit, named one of the best places to live in America by *Money* magazine, is an affluent suburb twenty miles from Manhattan, a haven for WASPs and Wall Street bankers who congregate at the many country clubs within its six square miles. We'd moved there in 1996 from Brooklyn, but even though it had been an ideal place to grow up, our family had never exactly fit in. In a neighborhood of white houses, my mom had chosen to paint our house a lavender-gray-purple, which prompted one of my sixth-grade classmates to comment: "My mom says that you're going to get polka dots too!" Eventually my mom changed the color to a less outrageous blue-gray.

Instead of relaxing into the nostalgia of being back in my childhood home, though, as I settled into the Summit house over the next few days I began to cling even more vehemently to the Manhattan life I'd left behind. On Sunday afternoon I became obsessed with filing an overdue article on a fairly simple story about a troupe of dancers that was opening off-Broadway who called themselves "Gimp," made up of disabled performers.

"They're not your typical dancers," I began. Unhappy with the line, I erased it. For the next half hour, I wrote, erased, and rewrote that same sentence until I gave up and began to pace, trying to wrestle myself out of writer's block. I wandered into the family room, where Mom and Allen were watching TV, desperate to tell them about my new trouble with words. But when I got there, I could no longer remember why I'd come.

The TV blasted the theme song to their favorite show, the medical drama *House*. Seconds later, the normally muted green of the couch grew noxiously garish.

Then the room seemed to pulsate and breathe, like the office hallway.

I heard my mom's voice, shrill and far away: "Susannah, Susannah. Can you hear me?"

Next thing I knew, my mom was sitting beside me on the couch, rubbing my feet, which had stiffened up in a painful charley horse. I looked up at her helplessly. She said, "I don't know what happened. It was like you were in a trance."

My mom and Allen exchanged worried glances and phoned Dr. Bailey to see if they could schedule an emergency appointment. The earliest he could do it, he said, was Monday.

I spent the weekend in Summit, ignoring calls from concerned coworkers and friends. I was too embarrassed by my own unexplainable behavior to talk to them and so consumed by the strange stirring in my mind that I turned away from those closest to me, which normally I would never have done. For some reason, I did pick up the phone once, when I saw it was my friend Julie, a *Post* photographer and the most carefree, lighthearted person I know. As soon as we started talking, I began to tell her everything: the seizures, the strange thoughts, the visions. Maybe it was because I knew her mother was a shrink. When I finished, it turned out that she had already spoken to her mother about me.

"She thinks it's possible that you're having a manic episode and that maybe you have bipolar disorder. Whatever it is, you should see a psychiatrist," she suggested.

Bipolar disorder. Even though it would have sounded grim at any other moment, now the idea was a relief. This made sense. A quick Google search revealed that the National Institute of Mental Health had a whole booklet dedicated to it: "a brain disorder that causes unusual shifts in moods" (yes); "often develops in a person's late teens or early adult years" (yes); "an overly joyful state is called a manic episode, an extremely sad or hopeless state is called a depressive episode" (yes and yes, which equals a mixed state). Another site listed at length the famous people who were suspected to suffer from bipolar disorder: Jim Carrey, Winston Churchill, Mark Twain, Vivien Leigh, Ludwig van Beethoven, Tim Burton. The list kept going and going. I was in good company. "No great mind has ever existed without a touch of madness," Aristotle said.

I spent the night in a state of ecstasy: I had a name for what plagued me, and those two words, which fell off the tongue so sweetly, meant everything. I didn't even want to be "cured." I now belonged to an exclusive club of creatives.

Unconvinced by my self-diagnosis, my mom and Allen drove me back to Dr. Bailey's office that Monday, March 16. The Miró painting no longer seemed as menacing. It matched my mood disorder. Dr. Bailey called us in almost immediately. His demeanor this time seemed far less jolly and grandfatherly, though overall he was pleasant. Again, he went through the basic neurological exam and wrote down "normal." Right then, I did feel normal. He jotted down notes on his pad as he asked me questions. Only later would I learn that he was missing details, writing down that I was "on a plane" when the first seizure occurred.

His tone was light when discussing the seizure, but then he slid his glasses down his nose, and suddenly sounded very serious. "Is your job very stressful?"

"Yes, I guess."

"Do you feel overwhelmed at times?"

"Sure."

"Tell me honestly," he said, as if preparing himself for me to let him in on a big secret. "There are no judgments here. How much alcohol are you drinking a day?"

I had to think about it. I hadn't had a drop of booze in the past week, but normally it helped me unwind, so I tended to have a sip of something most nights. "To be honest, about two glasses of wine a night. I usually split a bottle with my boyfriend, though he tends to drink more than I do." He made a note of this in his chart. I didn't understand that doctors usually doubled—even tripled—such numbers because patients often lie about their vices. Instead of two drinks a night, he probably believed the number was closer to six.

"Any drug use?"

"No. Not in years," I said, and quickly added, "I did some research on bipolar disorder, and I really think that's what I have."

He smiled. "I don't have any experience in this field, but it's a possibility. The receptionist will refer you to a very capable psychiatrist who will have more experience with these types of issues."

"Great."

"Okay, then. Well, otherwise, everything looks normal to me. I'm going to draw you up a prescription for Keppra, an anti-seizure medication. Take that, and everything should be fine. I'll see you in two weeks," he said and walked me to the waiting area. "I'm going to also have a little talk with your mother if you don't mind." He waved her into his office. After he had closed the door behind him, he turned to her.

"I think this is very simple. Plain and simple. She's partying too hard, not sleeping enough, and working too hard. Make sure she doesn't drink and takes the Keppra I prescribed, and everything should be fine."

My mom was filled with immense relief. It was just the answer she wanted to hear.

CHAPTER 10

MIXED EPISODES

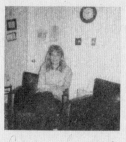

A llen drove us up to a prewar brownstone on the Upper East Side, where the psychiatrist, Sarah Levin, lived and worked. My mom and I walked to the entrance and pressed the buzzer. A Carol Kane falsetto trilled through the intercom: "Come right in and sit in the waiting area. I'll be right with you."

With its white walls, magazines, and bookcases filled with all the classics of literature, Dr. Levin's waiting area seemed straight out of a Woody Allen film. I was excited to see the psychiatrist. I wanted her to confirm, once and for all, my bipolar self-diagnosis, but also I considered psychiatric visits entertaining on a certain level. For a period of time after an old breakup, I had gone to three separate psychologists, testing them out. The exercise was largely self-indulgent, inspired by watching too many episodes of the HBO show *In Treatment*. First I saw the attractive young gay man who acted like my best friend and enabler; then a green and geeky (but cheap) shrink who took my insurance and immediately asked me about my relationship with my father; then an old curmudgeon who tried to hypnotize me with a plastic wand.

"Come on in," said Dr. Levin, appearing at the door. I smiled: she looked like Carol Kane too. She motioned for me to sit in the leather chair.

"I hope you don't mind, but I always take pictures of my patients to keep track of everyone," she said, nodding at the Polaroid camera in her hands. I posed, not sure if I should smile or remain serious. I remembered what my friend Zach from work had once told me years before when I first went on live television during the Michael Devlin affair: "Smile with your eyes." So that's what I tried to do.

"So tell me a bit about why you're here," she asked, cleaning her glasses.

"I'm bipolar."

"I'm sorry," she said. "Say that again?"

"I'm bipolar."

She nodded as if agreeing with me. "Are you on any medication for that?"

"No. I haven't been officially diagnosed. But I know. I mean, I know myself better than anyone, right? So I should know if I have it. And I know that I do," I rambled on, the illness imposing itself on my speech patterns.

She nodded again.

"Tell me why you think you're bipolar."

As I made my case through my strange, jumpy logic, she jotted down her impressions on two pages of wide-ruled paper: "Said she had bipolar disorder. Hard to conclude," she wrote. "Everything is very vivid. Started in last few days. Can't concentrate. Easily distracted. Total insomnia but not tired, not eating. Has grand ideas. No hallucinations. No paranoid delusions. Always impulsive."

Dr. Levin asked if I had any history of feeling this way and wrote, "She's had hypomanic attacks her whole life. Always has high energy. But has negative thoughts. She was never suicidal."

Dr. Levin's opinion was that I was experiencing a "mixed episode," meaning both manic and depressive elements typical of bipolar disorder. She moved several large books on her desk around until she found her scrip pad and scrawled out a prescription for Zyprexa, an antipsychotic prescribed to treat mood and thought disorders.

While I was in the office with Dr. Levin, my mother called my younger brother, a freshman at the University of Pittsburgh. Even though James was only nineteen, he already had a wise, old-soul quality that I've always found comforting.

"Susannah had a seizure," she told James, trying to control the wavering of her voice. James was stunned. "The neurologist is saying she drank too much. Do you think Susannah is an alcoholic?" my mom asked him.

James was adamant. "No way is Susannah an alcoholic."

"Well, Susannah's insisting that she's manic-depressive. Do you think that's a possibility?"

James thought on this for a moment. "No. Not in the least. That's just not Susannah. Sure, she can be excitable and temperamental, but she's not depressive. She's tough, Mom. We all know that. She deals with a lot of stress, but she handles it better than anyone I know. Bipolar doesn't make any sense to me."

"Me neither," my mom said. "Me neither."

CHAPTER 11
KEPPRA

Later that next night, I had an epiphany. Forget bipolar disorder: it was the antiseizure medication Keppra. The Keppra must be causing my insomnia, forgetfulness, anxiety, hostility, moodiness, numbness, loss of appetite. It didn't matter that I had been on the drug for only twenty-four hours. It was all the Keppra. An Internet search proved it. These were all side effects of that toxic drug.

My mother pleaded with me to take it anyway. "Do it for me," she begged. "Just please take the pill." So I did. Even during this time when I hardly recognize myself, there are still shadows of the real Susannah, a person who cares what her family and friends think, who doesn't want to cause them pain. Looking back, I think that's why, despite the battles, I often caved at my family's insistences.

That night, as the alarm clock by my bed struck midnight, I lifted my head with a start. *The damn pills. They're taking over my body. I'm going crazy. THE KEPPRA. I need it out of my system.* "*Throw it up, get it out!*" a voice chanted. I kicked off my sheets and jumped out of bed. *KEPPRA, KEPPRA.* I went to the hallway bathroom, ran the water, got on my knees, and knelt over the toilet bowl. I jammed my fingers down my throat, wiggling them around until I dry-heaved. I wiggled more. Thin white liquid. Nothing solid came up because I hadn't eaten in longer than I could remember. *DAMN KEPPRA.* I flushed the toilet, turned off the water, and paced.

The next thing I knew, I was upstairs on the third floor, where my mom and Allen slept. They'd moved up there when James and I were teenagers because it had worried them too much to hear us coming and going at night. Now I stood over my mom's bed and watched her sleep. The half-moon shone down on her. She looked so helpless, like a newborn baby. Swelling with tenderness, I leaned over and stroked her hair, startling her awake.

"Oh, my. Susannah? Are you okay?"

"I can't sleep."

She rearranged her mussed-up, cropped hair and yawned.

"Let's go downstairs," she whispered, taking my hand and leading me back into my bedroom. She lay down beside me, brushing out my tangled hair with her beautiful hands for over an hour until she fell back asleep. I listened to her breathing, soft and low, in and out, and tried to replicate it. But I didn't sleep.

The next day, on March 18, 2009, at 2:50 p.m., I wrote the first in a series of random Word documents that would become a kind of temporary diary over this period. The documents reveal my scattered and increasingly erratic thought processes:

> Basically, I'm bipolar and that's what makes me ME. I just have to get control of my life. I LOVE working. I LOVE it. I have to break up with Stephen. I can read people really well but I'm too jumbly. I let work take way too much out of my life.

During a conversation earlier that day when we discussed my future, I'd told my father that I wanted to go back to school, specifically to the London School of Economics, even though I had no history of studying business. Wisely, gently, my father suggested that I write down all my racing thoughts. So that's what I did for the next few days: "My father suggested writing in a journal, which is definitely helping me. He told me to get a puzzle and that was smart because he too thinks in puzzles (the way things fit together)."

Some of the statements are incoherent messes, but others are strangely illuminating, providing deep access to areas of my life that I'd never before examined. I wrote about my passion for journalism: "Angela sees something in me because she knows how hard it is to be good at this job, but that's journalism, it's a hard job. and maybe it's not for me I have a very powerful gut." And I went on about my need for structure in a life that was quickly falling to pieces: "Routine is important to me, as is discipline without it I tend to go a little bit haywire."

As I wrote these lines and others, I felt that I was piecing together, word by word, what was wrong with me. But my thoughts were tangled in my mind like necklaces knotted together in a jewelry box. Just when I thought I had untwisted one, I would realize it was connected to a rat's nest of others. Now, years later, these Word documents haunt me more than any unreliable memory. Maybe it's true what Thomas Moore said: "It is only through mystery and madness that the soul is revealed."

That night I walked into the family room and announced to my mom and Allen, "I've figured it out. It's Stephen. It's too much pressure. It's too much. I'm too young." My mom and Allen nodded empathetically. I left the room, but then, a few feet outside the doorway, another solution emerged. I retraced my steps. "Actually, it's the *Post*. I'm unhappy there, and it's making me crazy. I need to go back to school."

They nodded again. I left and then turned straight around again.

"No. It's my lifestyle. It's New York City. It's too much for me. I should move back to St. Louis or Vermont or someplace quiet. New York isn't for me."

By now they were staring at me, concern creasing their faces, but still they continued to nod accommodatingly.

I left once more, cantering from the family room to the kitchen and then back. This time I had it. This time I had figured it out. This time it all made sense.

The Oriental rug scraped my cheek.

Oval droplets of blood marring the pattern.

My mom's shrill screams.

I had collapsed on the floor, bitten my tongue, and was convulsing like a fish out of water, my body dancing in jerking motions. Allen ran over and put his finger in my mouth, but in a spasm I bit down hard on it, adding his blood to my own.

I came to minutes later to the sound of my mother on the phone with Dr. Bailey, frantic for some kind of answer. He insisted that I keep taking the medication and come in for an electroencephalogram (EEG) on Saturday, to test the electrical activity of my brain.

Two days later, that Friday, Stephen came to Summit to visit and suggested that we get out of the house and grab some dinner. He had been debriefed by my family about my deteriorating behavior and was on high alert, but he knew that it was important for me to leave the house (because of the threat of seizures, I could not drive a car) and maintain some semblance of an adult life. We headed to an Irish pub in Maplewood, New Jersey, where I had never been before. The bar was crowded with families and teenagers. People hovered around the hostess's desk, jockeying for reservations. I knew immediately that there were too many people. *They all stared at me. They whispered to each other, "Susannah, Susannah."* I could hear it. My breath got shallower, and I began to sweat.

"Susannah, Susannah," Stephen repeated. "She said it's a forty-minute wait. Do you want to wait or go?" He gestured to the hostess, who did in fact look at me curiously.

"Umm. Umm." *The old man who seemed to be wearing a toupee jeered at me.* The hostess raised her eyebrows. "Ummm."

Stephen grabbed my hand and walked me out of the restaurant into the freedom of the frigid air. Now I could breathe again. Stephen drove me to nearby Madison, to a dingy bar called Poor Herbie's where there was no wait. The waitress, a woman in her midsixties with frizzy bleached blond hair and gray roots, stood at the table with her left hand on her hip, waiting for our orders. I just stared at the menu.

"She'll take the chicken sandwich," Stephen said, after it was clear I was incapable of making such a momentous decision. "And I'll have the reuben."

When the food came, I could focus only on the greasy french dressing congealing on Stephen's corned beef sandwich. I looked down at my own sandwich despairingly; nothing could convince me to put it to my lips.

"It's too . . . grizzly," I told Stephen.

"But you didn't try it. If you don't eat this, there's nothing but gefilte fish and chicken livers at home," he joked, trying to lighten the mood by pointing out Allen's strange eating habits. Stephen finished his reuben, but I left the chicken sandwich untouched.

As we walked to the car, two conflicting urges struck me: I needed either to break up with Stephen here and now or profess my love to him for the first time. It could go either way; both impulses were equally intense.

"Stephen, I really need to talk to you." He looked at me oddly. I stammered, growing red before conjuring up the courage to speak, although I still didn't know what was going to come out of my mouth. He too was half-expecting me to break up with him at that moment. "I just. I just. I really love you. I don't know. I love you."

Tenderly he grasped my hands in his own. "I love you, too. You just have to relax." It was not how either of us had hoped this exchange would happen; it was not the kind of memory you recalled to your grandchildren, but there it was. We were in love.

Later that night, Stephen noticed that I had begun to steadily smack my lips together as if I was sucking on a candy. I licked my lips so often that my mom started to apply globs of Vaseline to keep them from cracking open and bleeding. Sometimes I would trail off midsentence, staring off into space for several minutes before continuing my conversation. During these moments, the paranoid aggression receded into a childlike state. These times

were the most unnerving for everyone, since I'd been pighead-
edly self-sufficient, even as a toddler. We didn't know it then, but
these too were complex partials, the more subtle types of seizures
that create those repetitive mouth movements and that foggy consciousness. I was getting worse by the day, by the hour even, but
no one knew what to do.

At 3:38 a.m., on March 21, as Stephen snored away upstairs,
I wrote again in my computer diary:

> Okay there's no place to start but you have to, ok? And don't
> be all "wow I didn't spell check this."

> I had the urge to baby stephen instead of allow him to baby me.
> I've been letting my parents baby me for too long.

> you have a mothering instinct (you held him in your arms). you
> felt you have untangled your mind when you are around him.
> you found your phone and remembered.

> talking to my father makes me feel more with it. my mom
> babies me way too much because she blames herself for the
> way I am. But she shouldn't. She's been a great mother. And she
> should know that.

> who gives a shit what anyone things about me. I'm going to

> Stephen: he keeps you sane. He's also very smart. Don't let how
> humble he is fool you, okay? You got this crossroads because
> of him and you should be forever grateful for that. So be kind
> to him.

Reading these entries now is like peering into a stranger's stream of consciousness. I don't recognize the person on the other end of the screen as me. Though she urgently attempts to communicate some deep, dark part of herself in her writing, she remains incomprehensible even to myself.

CHAPTER 12
THE RUSE

On Saturday morning, my mom tried to get me to return to Dr. Bailey's for the EEG. I had had two identifiable seizures and had developed an increasing number of worrying symptoms in the past week alone, and my family needed answers.

"Absolutely not," I grumbled, stamping my feet like a two-year-old. "I'm fine. I don't need this."

Allen walked outside to start the car as Stephen and my mother pleaded with me.

"Nope. Not going. Nope," I replied.

"We have to go. Please, just come," my mom said.

"Let me talk to her for a second," Stephen said to my mom, leading me outside. "Your mom is only trying to help you, and you're making her very upset. Will you please just come?"

I thought this over for a moment. I loved my mom. Fine. Yes. I would go. Then a moment later—No! I couldn't possibly leave. After a half hour more of persuading, I finally got into the back-seat of the car beside Stephen. As we drove out of our driveway and onto the street, Allen began to speak. I could hear him distinctly, though he wasn't moving his lips.

You're a slut. I think Stephen should know.

My whole body shook with anger, and I leaned threateningly toward the driver's seat. "What did you say?"

"Nothing," Allen said, sounding both surprised and exhausted.

That was the last straw. Swiftly, I unbuckled my seat beat, yanked open the car door, and prepared to jump out of the car headfirst. Stephen grabbed the back of my shirt in mid-leap, saving me from launching myself out of the vehicle. Allen slammed on the brakes.

"Susannah, what the hell are you doing?" my mom screamed.

"Susannah," Stephen said in a level tone, a timbre I had never before heard from him. "That is not okay."

Obedient again, I closed the door and crossed my arms. But hearing the *click* of the child's lock sent me into panic mode again. I flung myself against the locked door and screamed, "Let me out! Let me out!" over and over, until I was too exhausted to yell anymore, then rested my head against Stephen's shoulder and momentarily nodded off.

When I opened my eyes again, we had exited the Holland Tunnel and were entering Chinatown, with its sidewalk fish, swarms of tourists, and fake designer bag salesmen. The whole sordid scene disgusted me.

"I want coffee. Get me coffee. Now. I'm hungry. Feed me," I demanded, insufferably.

"Can't you wait until we get uptown?" my mom asked.

"No. Now." It suddenly seemed like the most important thing in the world.

Allen took a sharp turn, almost hitting a parked car, and took West Broadway to the Square Diner, one of the last authentic train car diners in New York City. Allen couldn't figure out how to unlock the child's lock, so I climbed over Stephen to get out of his door, hoping to disappear before any of them could catch up. Stephen suspected as much and followed me. Since I couldn't get away, I sauntered into the diner in search of coffee and an egg sandwich. It was Sunday morning, so the line to eat was long, but I wouldn't wait. I barbarously nudged an elderly lady out of my way and, spotting an open booth, sat down. I shouted obnoxiously to no one in particular, "I want coffee!"

Stephen took the seat opposite mine. "We can't stay. Can't you just get it to go?"

Ignoring him, I snapped my fingers, and the waitress arrived. "A coffee and egg sandwich."

"To go," Stephen added. He was mortified, rightly, by my behavior. I could be willful, but he had never seen me be rude.

Luckily the man behind the counter, who had been listening in on the exchange, called out, "I've got it." He turned his back to us and cooked the eggs. A minute later, he delivered a steaming cup of coffee and a cheese-covered egg sandwich in a brown paper bag. I swaggered out of the diner. The paper coffee cup was so hot that it burned my skin, but I didn't care. *I made things happen. I was powerful. When I snapped my fingers, people jumped.* If I couldn't understand what was making me feel this way, at least I could control the people around me. I threw the egg sandwich, uneaten, on the car floor.

"I thought you were hungry," Stephen said.

"I'm not anymore."

Mom and Allen exchanged glances in the front seat.

The traffic was light heading uptown, so we got to Dr. Bailey's quickly. When I walked into the office, something felt different about the place, odd, alien. I felt like Gonzo walking into the casino after he had dropped mescaline in *Fear and Loathing in Las Vegas*. Nothing was as it seemed, and everything dripped with apocalyptic meaning. The other waiting patients were caricatures, subhuman; the glass window that separated the receptionist from us seemed utterly barbaric; the Miró was smiling down at me again with that twisted, unnatural grin. We waited. It could have been minutes or several hours, I have no idea. Time didn't exist here. Eventually a middle-aged female technician called me into an examination room, wheeling in a cart behind her. She dug out a box full of electrodes and pasted all twenty-one of them, one by one, onto my scalp; first rubbing the dry skin, and then fixing them to my head with some kind of glue. She turned off the lights.

"Relax," she said. "And keep your eyes closed until I tell you to open them. Breathe deeply in and out. One complete breath for every two seconds."

She counted for me, one, two, exhale; one, two, exhale; one, two, exhale. And then faster, one, exhale; one, exhale; one, exhale. It went on forever. My face flushed, and I started to get dizzy and lightheaded. I heard her fiddling around with something across the room so I opened my eyes enough to see her handling a small flashlight.

"Open your eyes and look directly into the light," she said. It pulsated like a strobe, but with no apparent rhythm to its pattern. When she turned on the light to remove the electrodes, she began to speak to me.

"So are you a student?"

"No."

"What do you do?"

"I'm a reporter. I write for a newspaper."

"Stressful, huh?"

"Sure, I guess."

"There's nothing wrong with you," she said, gathering the electrodes back into the box. "I've seen this dozens of times, mostly with bankers and Wall Street guys who come in here all stressed out. There's nothing wrong with them; it's all in their heads." *It's all in my head.* When she closed the door behind her, I smiled. That smile turned into a laugh, a belly laugh dripping with bitterness and resentment. It all made sense. *This was all a ruse, set up to punish me for my bad behavior and tell me that I'm suddenly cured. Why would they try to trick me? Why would they arrange something this elaborate? She wasn't a nurse. She was a hired actor.*

My mother was the only person left in the waiting room; Allen had left to get the car, and Stephen, overwhelmed by my harrowing behavior on the ride in, had called his mom for consolation and advice. I gave my mom a wide, toothy smile.

"What's so funny?"

"Oh! You thought I wouldn't figure it out. Where's the mastermind?"

"What are you talking about?"

"You and Allen set this all up. You hired that woman. You hired everyone here. You told her what to say. You wanted to punish me. Well, it didn't work. I'm too smart for your tricks."

My mom's mouth fell open in horror, but my paranoia read it as nothing more than mock-surprise.

CHAPTER 13

BUDDHA

The whole time I'd been in Summit, I had been begging to return to my Manhattan apartment. I felt constantly under surveillance by my family. So on Sunday, the day after my EEG, my mom, exhausted by the week of sleepless nights and constant monitoring, agreed, against her better judgment, to let me revisit my apartment under one condition: I spend the night at my father's house. Though my behavior was worsening day by day, it was still difficult for her to reconcile the old image that she had of her daughter as trustworthy, hard working, and independent with the new, unpredictable, and dangerous one.

I quickly consented to spend the night with my father—I would have said anything to get back to my own studio. I felt calmer as soon as we arrived in Hell's Kitchen, being so close to freedom again. As soon as we saw my father and Giselle waiting outside on the front stoop of my building, I bounded out of the car. My mom and Allen didn't follow, but they did wait until the three of us were safely inside before driving away.

I was delighted to be back in my safe haven. Here was my cat, Dusty, a blue-haired stray who'd been tended by my friend Zach during my weeklong absence. I was even glad to see the unwashed clothes and black plastic bags filled with books and debris and the garbage overflowing with stale food. Home sweet home.

"What's that smell?" my father asked. I hadn't cleaned my apartment since the last time he came, and it had only gotten worse. Some of the leftover shrimp from the meal Stephen had cooked had spoiled in the garbage. Without hesitating, my father and Giselle began cleaning. They scrubbed the floors and disin-

fected every inch of that small apartment, but I didn't even offer
to help. I just walked around them, watching them clean and pre-
tending to gather my things.

"I'm so messy!" I said, stroking my cat triumphantly. "Messy,
messy, messy!"

After they finished, my father motioned for me to follow him
out of the apartment.

"Nah," I said, nonchalantly. "I think I'm just going to stay
here."

"Absolutely not."

"How about I meet you in Brooklyn after I get a few things
together?"

"Absolutely not."

"I will not leave!"

Dad and Giselle exchanged knowing glances, like they had prepared for such an outburst. Presumably Mom had warned them
about me. Giselle rounded up the cleaning supplies and headed
downstairs to get away from the unfolding unpleasantness.

"Come on, Susannah, we'll grab some coffee. I'll cook you dinner. It will be nice and calm. Just come over."

"No."

"Please. Will you do this for me?" he asked. It took a half
hour but finally I agreed, grabbing a handful of underwear and a
few other clean clothes. The illness seemed to wane momentarily,
allowing the old, reasonable Susannah to return briefly. The three
of us chatted a little as we walked toward the subway on Forty-
Second Street. But the calm didn't last long. Paranoia took hold as
I was crossing Ninth Avenue. *My father has taken my keys. I have
no way to get back to my apartment. I am his prisoner.*

"No. No. No!" I shouted in the middle of the street, stopping just as the lights turned green. "I'm not going. I want to go
home!" I felt my dad's tight grip on my shoulders as he pushed
me out of the way of the oncoming traffic. I continued to scream
as he hailed a cab. When the cab pulled up, he pushed me inside,
and Giselle entered on the other side so I was wedged between
them. They were determined to prevent another escape attempt.

"They're kidnapping me. Call the police! Call the police! They're taking me against my will!" I screamed at the Middle Eastern cab driver. He looked back in his rearview mirror but did not drive. "Let me go. I'm calling the cops!"

"Get out. Leave car. Now," the driver said.

My father gripped the bulletproof partition and said, through gritted teeth, "You better fucking drive. Don't you dare stop."

I can't imagine what the driver thought, because it must have looked tremendously suspicious, but he obliged. Soon he started to speed, darting in and out of traffic on the Brooklyn Bridge.

"I'm calling the police when I get out. You'll see. You'll be arrested for kidnapping!" I shouted at my dad. The driver glanced at us warily in the mirror.

"You do that," my dad said nastily. Giselle remained quiet and looked out the window, as if trying to block out the scene. Then my father softened his voice: "Why are you doing this? Why are you doing this to me?" Honestly, I had no idea. But I was convinced I wasn't safe in his care.

By the time we arrived at their brownstone in Brooklyn Heights, I was too exhausted to fight anymore. I had nothing left, which wasn't surprising since I hadn't eaten or slept in a week. When we got inside, Giselle and my father headed to the kitchen. They began to cook my favorite meal, penne arrabiata, as I sat on the couch in the living room, staring dazedly at my father's busts of Abraham Lincoln and George Washington. My father's house is an ode to American wars, filled with antiques and memorabilia spanning the Revolutionary War to World War II. He even calls one anteroom that separates the den from the living room the "war room." There are muskets from the Civil War; M1 Garands that were used from World War I to Vietnam; Colt revolvers from the 1800s; a Revolutionary War sword and a soldier's hat from the same era. Before the divorce, he'd kept most of these possessions in our Summit house's family room, which scared off many boyfriends during my high school years.

They set the long harvest table and brought over a heaping, pulsating dish of reds, greens, and yellows—tomato, basil, cheese, and penne—in a blue Le Creuset pot. Pancetta glistened unnaturally in the blood-red tomato sauce. I stifled the urge to vomit or throw the penne against the wall and just watched as my dad and Giselle ate the pasta in silence.

After dinner, I went into the kitchen to get some water. Giselle was cleaning. She walked past me to put the dishes in the sink, and as she moved, I heard her say, *"You're a spoiled brat."* The words hung in the air around me, like pockets of smoke. I didn't see her mouth move.

"What did you say to me?"

"Nothing," she said, looking surprised.

My father waited for me in his den in a patterned antique rocking chair that had belonged to his aunt. I opted for silence about what I believed Giselle had called me.

"Stay here with me tonight?" I asked him instead, sitting on the leather couch by his side. The TV was off, so we made small talk, our conversation punctuated by uneasy blocks of silence. "I'm scared of being alone."

"Of course," he said.

Then: "Leave me alone! Get out of the room."

And then, all over again: "I'm sorry. Will you please stay?"

This went on for several hours, moving from hysterics to accusations and then back to apologies. Beyond that, I can't remember much at all of that night, which might be my body's way of trying to preserve some self-respect. No one wants to think of herself as a monster. My father doesn't remember what happened either, although it's more likely that he has consciously chosen to forget. I do know that I said something terrible to him—something so awful that it made my father cry, the first time I had ever seen him cry in my life. But instead of generating sympathy, this just added to my twisted need for power. I ordered him to leave the room and go back upstairs to his bedroom.

A few moments later, a sickening blast and boom came from upstairs. *POUND POUND POUND*. I chose to ignore it.

I walked into his war room; picked up the Revolutionary War sword; removed it from its sheath, entranced by the blade; and then returned it. Then I heard Giselle's voice. *She was pleading with my father.* "Please don't hurt me," she begged. "Don't hurt me because of her."

Again, the imaginary *POUND POUND POUND.*

I returned to the den and sat back down on the leather couch. *A painting depicting the drafting of the Declaration of Independence bustled with activity. Over the fireplace, a large oil painting of a railroad scene came to life, the train emitting tufts of coal-covered smog. The bust of Lincoln seemed to follow me with its sunken eyes. The dollhouse that my father made for me when I was a child was haunted.*

POUND POUND POUND.

It was the sound of fists hitting a hard object, like a skull. I could see it all clearly. He was beating her because he was upset with me.

POUND POUND POUND.

I needed to find an exit. There had to be some way out. I clawed at the apartment door frantically but found it locked from the outside. *Is he keeping me in here to kill me next?* I hurled myself against the door, ignoring the shooting pains in my right shoulder. *I must get out. Let me out.*

"Let me out! Let me out! Someone help me!" I screamed, banging my fists against the door. I heard my father's heavy footsteps on the stairs above me. I ran. Where? Bathroom. I locked the door behind me and tried to move the heavy eight-foot armoire against the door to barricade myself in. The window. It overlooked a two-story drop; I figured I could survive the fall.

"Susannah, are you okay? Please open the door."

Yes, I could probably have made the jump. But then I caught sight of a small Buddha that Giselle kept on the bathroom counter. It smiled at me. I smiled back. Everything would be all right.

CHAPTER 14
SEARCH AND SEIZURE

Early the next morning, my mom and Allen arrived to pick me up. When I saw the Subaru, I bolted from my father's house.

"They kidnapped me. They held me against my will. Bad things are happening there. Drive," I commanded.

My father had already relayed the story of what had occurred overnight. After I had said those terrible things and insisted that he leave, he went upstairs to a room where he could monitor me through thin walls without my knowing. He tried to stay awake but nodded off. As soon as he heard me trying to break free, he ran downstairs to find me barricaded in the bathroom. It had taken him over an hour to coax me out and onto the couch, where he sat with me until dawn. He had called my mother, and they agreed that I needed to be admitted to the hospital. But they remained adamant about one thing: I would not be placed in a psychiatric ward.

Allen drove me straight back to Dr. Bailey's office as I rested in the backseat, once again resigned to my fate.

"Her EEG was completely normal," Bailey protested, looking through my file. "MRI normal, exam normal, blood work normal. It's all normal."

"Well, she's not normal," my mom snapped as I sat there, quiet and polite with my hands folded in my lap. She and Allen had made a pact that they would not leave Dr. Bailey's office without getting me admitted to a hospital.

"Let me put this as delicately as possible," the doctor said. "She's drinking too much, and she's exhibiting the classic signs of alcohol withdrawal." The symptoms matched: anxiety, depression, fatigue, irritability, mood swings, nightmares, headache,

insomnia, loss of appetite, nausea or vomiting, confusion, hallucinations, and seizures. "I know it's hard to hear about your own
daughter. But, really, there's nothing more I can say. She just has
to take the medication and knock off the partying," he said and
winked conspiratorially at me.

"Alcohol withdrawal?" My mother brandished a piece of red-
lined paper that she had prepared. "These are her symptoms: seizures, insomnia, paranoia, and it's all just getting worse. I haven't
seen her drink in over a week. She needs to be hospitalized, now.
Not tomorrow. Now."

He looked at me and back at her. He had no doubt he was
right but knew better than to argue. "I'll make some calls and see
what I can do. But I have to repeat: my feeling on this is that it's
a reaction to excessive alcohol consumption."

He left the office for a brief moment, returning with news.
"NYU has a twenty-four-hour EEG monitoring floor. Would you
be happy with that?"

"Yes," my mom said.

"They have a hospital bed ready this moment. I don't know
how long it will be open, so I would advise you to go to NYU
immediately."

"Great," she said, gathering her purse and folding her paper.
"We'll go right away."

We entered through revolving doors into the busy, recently remod-
eled lobby of New York University Langone Medical Center.
Nurses sprinted by in green scrubs, followed by nurses' assistants
in purple scrubs; doctors in white lab coats chatted at the cross-
roads of the corridors; the patients, some with bandages, some on
crutches, some in wheelchairs, some on gurneys, journeyed past,
dead-eyed and unspeaking. There was no way I belonged *here*.

We found our way to Admitting, which was a group of chairs
surrounding a small desk, where a woman dispatched patients to
different floors across the gigantic hospital.

"I want coffee," I said.

My mother looked annoyed. "Really? Now? Fine. But be back right away." A part of my mom believed the old, responsible me was still in there somewhere, and she simply trusted that I wouldn't escape. Luckily, this time she was right.

A small stand nearby sold coffee and baked goods. I calmly chose a cappuccino and a yogurt.

"What do you have on your mouth?" my mother asked when I returned. "And why are you smiling like that?"

The strange taste of foam, a mixture of saliva and steamed milk, on my upper lip.

White lab coats.

The hospital's cold floor.

"She's having a seizure!" My mom's voice echoed across the vast hallway as three doctors descended on my shaking body.

From here on, I remember only very few bits and pieces, mostly hallucinatory, from the time in the hospital. Unlike before, there are now no glimmers of the reliable "I," the Susannah I had been for the previous twenty-four years. Though I had been gradually losing more and more of myself over the past few weeks, the break between my consciousness and my physical body was now finally fully complete. In essence, I was gone. I wish I could understand my behaviors and motivations during this time, but there was no rational consciousness operating, nothing I could access anymore, then or now. This was the beginning of my lost month of madness.

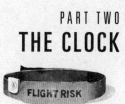

What is today's date?
Who is the President?
How great a danger do you pose, on a scale of one to ten?
What does "people who live in glass houses" mean?
Every symphony is a suicide postponed, true or false?
Should each individual snowflake be held accountable for the avalanche?
Name five rivers.
What do you see yourself doing in ten minutes?
How about some lovely soft Thorazine music?
If you could have half an hour with your father, what would you say to him?
What should you do if I fall asleep?
Are you still following in his mastodon footsteps?
What is the moral of "Mary Had a Little Lamb"?
What about his Everest shadow?
Would you compare your education to a disease so rare no one else has
    ever had it, or the deliberate extermination of indigenous populations?
Which is more puzzling, the existence of suffering or its frequent absence?
Should an odd number be sacrificed to the gods of the sky, and an even
    to those of the underworld, or vice versa?
Would you visit a country where nobody talks?
What would you have done differently?
Why are you here?

FRANZ WRIGHT, *"Intake Interview," Wheeling Motel*

CHAPTER 15

THE CAPGRAS DELUSION

PURPOSE OF CONSULTATION (include diagnosis at time of request): *psychosis* *(seen by C-L)*
Mocell 908451 2972; W 212 375-8952   prn haldol, geodon
24 yo BHF h/o melanoma presents with numbness of L side 1 month ago, now
with 5 seizures in last 3 days. On interview pt with labile mood, inappropriate
affect at times tangential, belief that father turned into someone else to play trick on her,
unclear if hallucinating. Pt had taken Keppra prior to admission, duration unclear, but
stopped on own due to irritability. MRI in 2/09 normal.   3/24 GTc = 472

I was admitted in midafternoon on March 23, ten days after that first blackout while watching the PBS show with Gwyneth Paltrow. The NYU Langone Medical Center has one of the largest epilepsy units in the world, but the only bed available on the eighteen-patient floor was in the advanced monitoring unit (AMU), a four-person room dedicated to "grid patients," people with severe epilepsy who need electrodes implanted in their brains so that the center can record the electrical activity required before some types of epilepsy surgery. Occasionally other patients, like me, ended up here due to lack of space. The room has its own nurses' station, where a staff member monitors the patients twenty-four hours a day. Two cameras hang above each bed, constantly surveying every patient on the floor so that the hospital can have physical as well as electrical evidence of seizures (when a patient is discharged, most of the footage is discarded; the hospital keeps only the seizure events and abnormal circumstances). All of this surveillance would prove essential to me later, when I began to try to reconstruct what happened to me during these lost weeks.

After my seizure in the lobby's admitting area, my mother and stepfather trailed behind the gurney as the medic team wheeled me onto the epilepsy floor. Two different nurses then brought me into the AMU. Diverted by their new roommate, the room's three other patients quieted when I arrived. The nurse practitioner took down my health history, noting that I was cooperative with just a hint of delay, which she figured was related to the aftermath of the seizure. When I was unable to answer questions, my mother, clutching her folder full of documents, answered in my stead.

The nurses settled me onto a bed that had two precautionary side guardrails; the bed itself was lowered as close as possible to the ground. Nurses began to arrive approximately once an hour to get my vitals: blood pressure, pulse, and the results of a basic neurological exam. My weight was on the low side of normal, my blood pressure high-normal, and my pulse slightly accelerated but not alarmingly so, given the circumstances. The assessments, which covered everything from bowel movements to level of consciousness, were all normal.

An EEG technician interrupted the screening, pulling a cart behind him. He began unloading handfuls of the multicolored electrodes—reds, pinks, blues, and yellows—like the ones from my EEG at Dr. Bailey's office. The wires fed into a small, gray EEG box, similar in shape and size to a wireless Internet router, which connected to a computer that would record my brain waves. These electrodes measure the electrical activity along the scalp, tracking the chatter of electrically charged neurons and translating their actions as waves of activity.

As the technician began to apply the adhesive, I stopped cooperating. It took him half an hour to place the twenty-one electrodes as I squirmed. "Please, stop!" I insisted, thrashing my arms as my mother caressed my hands, trying ineffectually to calm me. I was acting even more mercurial than in recent days. Things seemed to be going downhill fast.

Eventually my tantrum receded, but I continued to cry as the smell of fresh glue permeated the air. The tech finished applying the wires and, before he left, handed me a small pink backpack that looked as if it belonged to a preschooler. It held my little "Internet router," which would allow me to walk around but remain connected to the EEG system.

It was already clear that I would not be an easy patient, given the way I screamed at visitors and lashed out at nurses during those first few hours on the floor. When Allen arrived, I pointed and yelled at him, insisting that the nurses "get this man out of my room." Similarly, I loudly accused my dad of being a kidnapper when he arrived, and I demanded that they bar him as well. Because I was still in the midst of what seemed to be psychosis, many tests were impossible to conduct.

Later that evening, an on-call neurologist came to conduct a second basic health history. Immediately she noticed that I was "labile," meaning prone to mood swings, and "tangential," meaning that I skipped from topic to topic without clear transitions. Nonetheless, I did manage to describe my history of melanoma before I began to grow so illogical that the interview had to be postponed.

"So what year was it that you were diagnosed?" the neurologist asked.

"He's playing a trick on me."

"Who's playing a trick on you?"

"My dad."

"What do you mean?"

"He's changing into people. He's turning into different people to play tricks on me."

The neurologist wrote "unclear if hallucinating" on her consultation form and prescribed a low-dose of the antipsychotic drug Geodon, often used to treat the symptoms of schizophrenia. She put in a request for a member of the psychiatric team to perform a closer examination.

Not only did I believe that my family members were turning into other people, which is an aspect of paranoid hallucinations, but I also insisted that my father was an imposter. That delusion has a more specific name, Capgras syndrome, which a French psychiatrist, Joseph Capgras, first described in 1923 when he encountered a woman who believed that her husband had become a "double." For years, psychiatrists believed this syndrome was an outgrowth of schizophrenia or other types of mental illnesses, but more recently, doctors have also ascribed it to neurobiological causes, including brain lesions. One study revealed that Capgras delusions might emerge from structural and circuitry complications in the brain, such as when the parts of the brain responsible for our interpretations of what we see ("hey, that man with dark hair about 5'10", 190 pounds looks like my dad") don't match up with our emotional understanding ("that's my dad, he raised me"). It's a little like déjà vu, when we feel a strong sense of intimacy and familiarity but it's not connected to anything we actually have experienced before. When these mismatches occur, the brain tries to make sense of the emotional incongruity by creating an elaborate, paranoid fantasy ("that looks like my dad, but I don't *feel* like he's my dad, so he must be an imposter") that seems to come straight out of *The Invasion of the Body Snatchers*.

EEG video, March 24, 1:00 a.m., 6 minutes

I am sleeping in bed, wearing a green and brown striped T-shirt and a white cotton hat. The ivory bedsheets are pulled up to my throat, and the cushioned guardrails are at their highest level, making the bed look, from above, like an adult-sized bassinet. I sleep in a fetal position, clutching my pillow. In a moment or two, I awake; fiddle with my cap, looking upset; and pull at the patient ID band on my right hand, folding my arms over my chest. I grab for my cell phone. End of tape.

I need to pee. I snatch up my pink backpack and unplug the cord and head to the shared bathroom. As I lower my black leggings and my underwear to my knees, I can't shake the feeling that I'm being watched. I look to my right, and a big brown eye peers in at me from a slit in the door.

"Get the fuck away from me!"

I cover my private parts, lift my pants, and sprint back to bed, pulling the covers to my eyes. I call my mom.

"They're trying to hurt me. They're making fun of me. They're putting shots in my arm," I whisper, trying to keep my voice low enough so that the other three patients and the nurse manning the in-room station can't hear me.

"Susannah, please try to stay calm. I promise you no one is try-ing to hurt you," my mom says.

"They're spying on me. They watch me when I go to the bath-room."

She pauses before speaking again. "Is this true?"

"How can you ask me that? Do you think I'd make it up?"

"I'm going to talk to them about this," she says, her voice growing frenzied.

"Do you think they'll tell you, 'Yeah, we're abusing your daughter'? Do you think they'll admit that?"

"Are you sure this is happening, Susannah?"

"Yes."

I hang up on her as I hear the shuffling of feet. A nurse walks near my bed. "Please don't use the phone with the EEG equip-ment. It interferes. And it's late. Everyone is sleeping."

Then she whispers, softly, tauntingly, without moving her lips, "I see you on the news."

"What did you say?"

"Why you no let your father in? He's a good man," the nurse says, her voice wafting around me like a vapor until she disap-pears behind the curtain.

Everyone is out to get me. I'm not safe here. I look up at the video cameras. They are watching me. If I don't leave now, I will never get out alive. I grab a handful of electrodes and pull. A patch of hair comes out with it, but no pain registers. Absently, I stare at the virgin roots of my dyed blond hair and then reach for more.

That night, I dashed out of the hospital room and into the hall-way, where a group of nurses caught up to me and returned me to the AMU room as I battled ferociously, kicking and screaming. It was my first, but not my last, attempt at escape.

CHAPTER 16

POSTICTAL FURY

Deborah Russo, an attending neurologist on the epilepsy floor, visited me on the second day to conduct yet another examination. She came during the morning shift, accompanied by doctors, nurses, and a few med students. They were "the team." Knowing about my escape attempt the night before, Dr. Russo sized up the room and confirmed that all seizure precautions were being maintained before moving on to the basic neurological exam: "touch your nose, stick out your tongue," etc. I interrupted her midreview.

"You need to let me out of here. I don't belong here," I confided, looking nervous. "They're all saying bad things about me."

"Who's talking to you?"

"The people on the TV."

Dr. Russo allowed me to ramble on for a few minutes before redirecting me. "Can you tell me a little about how you felt before you came to the hospital?"

"I felt like I disappeared."

"Can you explain what that means?"

"It felt like I was tired. I was tired until today."

Russo wrote down "too tangential and disorganized to give us a full history" and continued with her exam. "I'm going to ask you some basic questions, and you do your best to answer them, okay? What is your name?"

"Susannah," I said, craning my neck toward the TV set.

"What year is it?"

"You don't hear that? They're talking about me. Look, look, they're talking about me right now."

"Susannah, would you try to answer my questions?" Dr. Russo said, motioning for a nurse to turn off the television set. "What year is it?"

"2009."

"Who is the president?"

"Obama."

"Where are you?"

"I need to get out of here. I need to leave. I need to go."

"I understand. But where are you right now?"

"The hospital," I answered, caustically. Dr. Russo moved on, shining a light into my pupils with a small flashlight, checking for constriction and eye movement. All normal.

"Susannah, please smile for me."

"No more. I don't want to do this anymore," I said.

"It won't take long."

"I want out now!" I screamed, launching myself off the bed. The team waited out my outburst, but even once I was calm again, I continued to pace, tugging at my EEG leads and lunging toward the door. "Let me out of here!" I snarled at the team, trying to push my way out of the room. "Let me go home!"

Dr. Russo led me back to the bed several times, calling for the help of a nurse's assistant. She green-lighted a dose of Haldol, an antipsychotic. Later, typing up her impressions at the nurses' station, she wrote that the "patient appears to be manic and psychotic." She had two possible diagnoses: "First presentation of bipolar, versus postictal psychosis." "Ictal" means seizure, so post-ictal psychosis is psychotic behavior following a cluster of seizures. PIP, as it's called, can persist for as little as twelve hours or as long as three months, but the mean is about ten days. In 1838 a French psychiatrist described the condition as "postictal fury." A quarter of psychotic people treated in epilepsy wards suffer from PIP.

Later that morning, the third doctor, William Siegel, arrived alone. He introduced himself to me and then to my mother, who was already aware of his stellar reputation. A day earlier, she had mentioned his name to her general practitioner, who had said:

"You got Siegel? How did you pull that off?" Siegel was charismatic and approachable. After the neurological exam, he extended his hand to my mother and said, "We will figure this out. Susannah will be fine." My mother clung to these words like a life raft and nicknamed the doctor "Bugsy"—her own doctor gangster.

CHAPTER 17

MULTIPLE PERSONALITY DISORDER

The mind is like a circuit of Christmas tree lights. When the brain works well, all of the lights twinkle brilliantly, and it's adaptable enough that, often, even if one bulb goes out, the rest will still shine on. But depending on where the damage is, sometimes that one blown bulb can make the whole strand go dark.

The day after we met Dr. "Bugsy," Dr. Sabrina Khan from the Department of Psychiatry arrived and introduced herself to Stephen and me. She was the fourth doctor to join the team and had already heard about my two escape attempts: one in the early morning and one this afternoon with Dr. Russo. In her progress note, Dr. Khan described me as slightly disheveled and fidgety, wearing "revealing pajamas" (my tight leggings and a see-through white shirt) and playing with my dangling EEG leads. It was important for her to provide a visual picture to match the psychological one, because my rumpled, suggestive appearance could be a sign of mania: those on a high often forgo grooming and exhibit less impulse control, engaging in destructive acts like sexual promiscuity. Though I had no previous history of mental illness, I was within the age range for psychotic breaks, which tend to occur in the late teens or early twenties, but also frequently happen later in life for women.

While she was writing, I announced, unprompted, "I have multiple personality disorder."

Dr. Khan nodded patiently. I had picked one of the most controversial diagnoses in the field of psychiatry. Now called dissociative identity disorder (DID), it is a condition where a person exhibits several distinct and entirely separate identities, to the point that the patient is often unaware of the other "selves." Some doctors believe it exists, and others do not (especially in light of news that its poster child, Sybil, was a fraud). Many patients conflate DID with other types of mental illnesses, like schizophrenia. In any case, I was clearly confused.

"Have you been diagnosed by any psychiatrist or psychologist in the past?" she asked gently.

"Yes. A psychiatrist said I had bipolar disorder."

"And were you taking any medication for that?"

"I refused to take it. I spit it out. I need out of here. I don't belong here. I belong in a psychiatric ward. I belong in Bellevue. It's not safe for me here."

"Why is it not safe for you here?"

"Everyone is talking about me. They're all talking about me and making fun of me behind my back. I belong in Bellevue where they can take care of my disorder. I don't know why I'm here. I can hear what the nurses are saying about me. I can hear their thoughts, and they aren't saying nice things."

Dr. Khan wrote down "paranoid ideation."

"You can hear their thoughts?" she repeated.

"Yes. The whole world is making fun of me."

"What else can you hear?"

"The people on the TV are talking about me too."

Dr. Khan wrote "ideas of reference," a patient's belief that newspaper articles, songs, or TV shows refer directly to him or her. "Do you have any history of family members with mental illness?"

"I don't know. My grandmother might have had bipolar disorder. But they're all crazy." I laughed. Then I turned on her. "You know that I have the right to sign myself out, right? I can walk out of here. I can't legally be held here against my will. I don't want to talk anymore."

Dr. Khan wrote down her differential diagnoses, which included "Mood Disorder, not otherwise specified" and "Psychotic Disorder, not otherwise specified." She was concerned that, in light of the seizures and my history of melanoma, they should be looking for neurological causes.

If there was no underlying disease that could explain my sudden psychosis, she suggested bipolar I as a possible explanation. Bipolar I is a mood disorder characterized by a manic or mixed (both manic and depressive) episode. On a scale from 1 (most dire cases) to 100 (no symptoms), I received a score of 45, which translated to "serious symptoms." Dr. Khan recommended that the staff assign me a security guard, called a one-to-one, to try to prevent future escape attempts.

I can't hear their voices anymore. Her skin is so smooth. I stare at the doctor's cheekbones and pretty olive skin. I stare harder, harder, harder still. Her face swirls before me. Strand by stand her hair turns gray. Wrinkles, first just around her eyes, and then around her mouth and across her cheeks, now line her entire face. Her cheeks sink in, and her teeth turn yellow. Her eyes begin to droop, and her lips lose their shape. The striking young doctor ages right before my eyes.

I turn away and look at Stephen, who stares back at me. Stephen's stubble morphs from brown into a muted gray; his hair turns white like snow. He looks like his father. Out of the corner of my eye, I watch the doctor. Now she is growing more radiant with each passing second. All the wrinkles on her face smooth out, her eyes grow pert and oblong, her cheeks gain baby fat, and her hair turns a deep chestnut brown. She's thirty, twenty, thirteen.

I have a gift. I can age people with my mind. This is who I am. And they cannot take this away from me. I am powerful. Stronger than I have ever been in my life.

CHAPTER 18
BREAKING NEWS

Later that same day, a fifth doctor joined the team. My case had piqued the interest of Dr. Ian Arslan, a psychopharmacologist who topped six feet and who looked more like an aging hippie than a doctor. Because of his fondness for beat generation writers and his cerebral way of communicating abstract medical jargon, a colleague described him as a "walking beatnik dictionary."

He had already heard about my escape attempts and paranoid delusions, so he approached my mother first, asking her to walk him through the past few weeks of my bizarre behavior. Then he interviewed my father. After a short interview with me, which yielded a vivid portrait of my dysfunction, he gathered statements from the nursing staff and even called up Dr. Bailey, who, according to Arslan's notes, told him that I "drank excessively up to two *bottles* of wine per night." Dr. Bailey's estimate of my vices seemed to have substantially increased. Having summarized all of this, Dr. Arslan jotted down the two diagnoses he wanted to rule out: postictal psychosis and schizoaffective disorder. Knowing it would upset them, he did not share the second diagnosis with my parents.

The term *schizoaffective disorder* was introduced in 1933 in a much-quoted paper, "The Schizoaffective Psychoses": "Like a bolt from the blue, full-blown delusions suddenly shatter the poise of a fully rational mind . . . and flare up without premonitory signs. . . ."

A more updated description defines it as a diagnosis when mood symptoms, which are characteristic of bipolar disorder, overlap with psychosis, which is symptomatic of thought disorders like schizophrenia. The American Psychiatric Association's *Diagnostic and Statistical Manual of Mental Disorders,* version IV-TR, the edition that was used during my hospital stay, defines the disorder as an "uninterrupted period of illness during which, at some time, there is either a Major Depressive Episode, a Manic Episode, or a Mixed Episode." To earn such a diagnosis, a patient has to experience two or more of the following: positive symptoms, like delusions, hallucinations, and disorganized speech, and negative symptoms, such as mutism or general apathy.

EEG video, March 24, 11:06 p.m., 11 minutes

"Patient push button in room 1279. Patient push button in room 1279," the prerecorded voice says. My hospital gown peeks through from the covers that are pulled up to my neck, and I hold a cell phone to my ear, talking animatedly into its mouthpiece. It is unclear if anyone is on the other end. I pick up the hospital-provided TV remote and speak into it. There is certainly no one at the other end of that conversation. I point to the camera accusingly, gesticulating wildly, and put my hands to my head in frustration.

"Oh my god," I cry and hit the nurses' call button.

"Can I help you?" a nurse says over the intercom.

"No, no, it's okay."

"Ma'am? Lady? Miss? I'm coming," another nurse chimes in.

I'm mumbling to myself now. "I don't know what's happening. I'm going to turn my phone off." I toss my cell phone to the foot of the bed. A nurse arrives with some pills, and I swallow them without hesitation, like I'm taking a shot of tequila. "I can't have it on me. I'm on the news."

The nurse answers, but too softly for the video to pick it up.

I begin to shout and kick my legs, and I grab for the nurse's call button. "Please, please, please. I'm freaking out, I'm freaking out."

"Patient push button in room 1279. Patient push button in room 1279."

"Please put the TV back on. PLEASE PUT THE TV BACK ON!"

Ignoring my outburst, the nurse positions the guardrails to make sure they're firmly in place.

"Don't you see? I'm on TV, I'm on the news," I howl. I pick up the TV remote and speak into it again. And then place my head in my hands and rock back and forth. "Please, please, please. Oh my god, oh my god. Please get me a doctor. Please get me a doctor. Please, please, please."

The nurse leaves. There is a flushing of toilets. I stare straight up at the ceiling as if I am praying.

End of video.

"We'll be investigating what's happening with news reporter Susannah Cahalan, currently at New York University," a coiffed female anchor announces. I am top-of-the-hour news.

"I'm on the news!" I call out. Nobody answers.

"Her father was recently arrested for the murder of his wife," the anchor says as the camera pans to my father walking hand-cuffed through a sea of paparazzi, bulbs flashing, and reporters with their notebooks open and ready to lunge.

I've been so stupid. I shouldn't have answered calls from coworkers. They are secretly writing down what I'm saying. They know I cried in the newsroom. They'll put that into my story. "New York Post Reporter Unravels after Father Kills Wife."

"I'm on the news!" I grab the emergency nurse's call button. They have to know about the plot. They have to know not to let anyone in. "They're all going to try to interview me," I scream into my cell phone. Beads of sweat form on my brow. I wipe them away.

I hear the cackling of the patient to my left, a South American woman who spent all day chatting with her visitors in Spanish—or was it Portuguese? Now she's laughing at me. Maybe she was laughing at me the whole time. I hear her fake fingernails tap her cell phone keys. She's still speaking in Spanish, or whatever language it is, but now I can understand it.

"There's a girl from the New York Post in the bed next to me.

I'm going to record her with my cell phone and I'll give you all the information and you can give it to the Post. *Tell them it's an exclusive from someone in the hospital." She laughs again.*

"This girl is loco, trust me. Trust me, this is good stuff, I promise. We can make a lot of money with this scoop. Ca-ha-ha. Call all the local stations. I'll tell them everything. Just make sure we get some money out of it. Ca-ha-ha."

PSSSSTTTTT

What the hell was that?

PSSSSSTTTT

I hear it again.

PSSSTTTT *over here.*

I turn my head to the left. The South American woman has stopped her maniacal texting and has moved the curtain with her hand so that I can see her face.

"The nurses here are bad news," *she says softly.*

"What?" *I ask, not sure if I heard her correctly or if she spoke at all.*

"Shhhh, they can hear you," *she hisses, pointing to the cameras.* "The nurses here aren't right. I don't trust any of them."

Yes, yes, Strange Spanish Lady, that is true. But why is this undercover agent telling me this? She moves the curtains back in place, leaving me alone.

I need to leave. Now. Once again I grab the wires on my head, handful by handful, pulling them out with chunks of hair, and throw them on the floor. Instantly, I'm at the door. I'm through it. My heart pounds. I can feel it leaping up into my lungs. The security guard doesn't notice me. I sprint to the red EXIT sign. A nurse runs up beside me. Think, think, think, Susannah. I dodge into a hallway and run, racing, racing, racing—directly into another nurse's arms.

"Let me go home! Let me leave!"

She takes me by the shoulder. I kick her, screaming. I bite at the air. I must leave. I must go. LET ME GO. The cold floor. A purple lady grabs hold of my feet as the other nurse holds my arms down. "Please, please," I try to say through clenched teeth. "Please let me go."

Darkness.

Interval History

Interval History:

Patient became very agitated last evening. She ripped off her electrodes, and ran past 1:1 up and down hallways. This occurred despite receiving Seroquel. She was then given Ativan for agitation, and placed temporarily in a chest posey for safety by on call resident. She also received 25 mg Lopressor yesterday early evening for elevated BP and tachycardia. Vitals were ordered Q4h.

CHAPTER 19

BIG MAN

Two escape attempts earned me a one-to-one guard; now, after the third attempt in as many days, one nurse casually suggested to my father that if I kept dislocating the wires and trying to escape, I wouldn't be allowed to stay. "If she doesn't stop with that behavior, she'll be moved to a place that won't have this level of care. And she won't like the place as much, I can promise you that," she told him. My dad heard the threat loud and clear: if I continued along this path, I would be sent to a psychiatric ward. He decided that whatever happened, he would be by my side. He and I hadn't spent much time together since the divorce, and he was making up for it now. Having just left his banking job, he had the freedom and flexibility to spend his days with me. And he wanted the staff to know someone was looking out for me. He knew people often saw him as intimidating—despite his average height and build, my babysitter Sybil had always called him "big man"—and he was determined to capitalize on this if it would help me. Since I wouldn't let him in the room, still convinced he'd murdered Giselle, he decided to hold his vigil out in the hall and read a book.

In the interim, Dr. Russo had changed the chief complaint in her daily progress note from "seizures" to "psychosis and possible seizures" and then finally to just "psychosis." Postictal psychosis had become less of a primary diagnosis because I had not had a seizure since admission. In those with PIP, the psychosis is unlikely to continue unabated or increase in intensity without any seizure activity. Tests for hyperthyroidism, which can cause psychosis, came back negative, but they had to hold off on other tests. I was still far too psychotic for any more invasive examinations.

However, Dr. Russo also added a line in her progress note that had not been there before: "Transfer to psych [ward], if psych team feels this is warranted." Like Dr. Arslan, she chose not to tell my parents about this new suggestion.

```
she ll need to leave the floor for the
study.  Continue 1:1.  Transfer to psych
if psych team feels this is warranted.
Psychosis management per psychiatry,
appreciate input.
```

Although many of these findings were kept from my family and me, it was clear that my place on the epilepsy floor was becoming more and more precarious, just as the nurse had warned my father, both because my seizures seemed to have stopped and because I was such a difficult patient. Sensing that attitudes toward me improved and the level of care rose when company arrived, my dad stuck to his promise and started to arrive first thing every morning. Alone, I could not fight this battle.

My mother came every day, during her lunch hours, any breaks she could get from work, and then again after 5:00 p.m. She maintained several running lists of questions, lobbing one after another at the doctors and nurses, relentless even as so many of her questions remained unanswerable. She collected detailed notes, writing down doctors' names, home numbers, and unfamiliar medical terms she planned to look up. Though they were barely on speaking terms, she and my father also established a journal system so that they could communicate developments with each other when the other was absent. Though it had been eight years since their divorce, it was still hard for them to be in the same room with each other, and this shared journal allowed them to maintain common ground in the shared fight for my life.

Stephen too played a primary emotional role. I'm told that I would visibly relax when he arrived in the room carrying a leather briefcase that was often filled with *Lost* DVDs and nature documentaries for us to watch together. The second night I was there, though, I clutched his hand and said, "I know this is too much for you. I understand if you don't come back. I understand if I never see you again." It was then, he later told me, that he made a pact with himself not unlike my parents': if I were in the hospital, he would be there too. No one had any idea if I'd ever be myself again, or if I'd even survive this. The future didn't matter—he cared only about being there for me as long as I needed him. He would not miss even one day. And he didn't.

The fourth day, doctors number six, seven, eight, and nine joined the team: an infectious disease specialist who reminded my dad of his uncle Jimmy, who had earned the Purple Heart after storming the beaches of Normandy in World War II; an older, gray-haired rheumatologist; a soft-spoken autoimmune specialist; and an internist, Jeffrey Friedman, a spritely man in his early fifties who, despite the severity of the situation, exuded a natural optimism.

Dr. Friedman, who had been summoned to address my high blood pressure, was immediately sympathetic. He had daughters my age. When he walked into the room, he found me unkempt and confused, fidgeting in bed as Stephen, who sat by my side, tried in vain to calm me. I seemed both sluggish and frantic.

Dr. Friedman attempted a basic health history, but I was too paranoid and preoccupied with those "watching me" to talk coherently, so he went ahead and measured my blood pressure. He was alarmed: with a blood pressure reading at 180/100, those numbers alone could cause brain bleeding, stroke, or death. *If she were a computer,* he thought, *we would have to restart her hard drive.* He recommended placing me immediately on two different blood pressure medications.

As Dr. Friedman left the room, he identified my dad outside, sitting in the waiting area reading a book. As the two men chatted about what I was like before I'd gotten sick, my father described me as an active kid, a straight A student who made friends easily, who played hard and worked hard. That picture contrasted sharply with the disarrayed young woman Dr. Friedman had just examined. Even so, he looked my dad directly in his eyes and said, "Please stay positive. It will take time, but she will improve." When Dr. Friedman embraced him, my dad broke down, a brief surrender.

CHAPTER 20

THE SLOPE OF THE LINE

In the few weeks since my strange symptoms had begun, my dad had been spending much more time with me than usual. He was determined to support me as much as possible, but it was taking a toll on him; he had withdrawn from the rest of his life, even from Giselle. Since my breakdown in his apartment, he had also started keeping a daily journal, independent of the one he shared with my mom, not only to try to help him piece together the medical developments but also simply to help himself cope. After my second escape attempt, he wrote a heartbreaking entry about praying that God would take him instead of me.

He remembers in particular one cold, damp, early spring morning, driving to the hospital with Giselle in silence. He knew she would have given anything to help share some of his suffering, but even so, he remained disengaged, bottling up his anguish the way he always had.

At the hospital, he kissed Giselle good-bye and squeezed onto the crowded elevator. It was excruciating taking this trip alongside the fresh-faced new fathers being ferried to the maternity floor, some of whom bounded vigorously off the elevator. Life was just beginning for these people. The next stop was the cardiac floor, full of concerned looks, and then finally it was the twelfth floor: epilepsy. His turn to get off.

As he walked past a wing under renovation, he caught the eye of a middle-aged construction worker, who quickly looked to the floor in embarrassment. Good things were not happening on twelve; everyone knew that. For the past three days, while spending his hours in the temporary, makeshift waiting room, he had been taking stock of the neighboring activity. One particularly sad story was occurring just across the hall, where a young man was recovering after falling down a shaft and sustaining a massive head injury. His elderly parents came every day to see him, but no one seemed hopeful about his recovery. My dad said a quick prayer, pleading with God that my fate would be different from that young man's, and he breathed deeply as he prepared himself to see what state I was in this morning. I had just been moved to a new, private room, which seemed like a step in the right direction. On his way to my room, he noticed another patient beckoning him over.

"Is that your daughter?" the woman asked, motioning toward my room.

"Yes."

"I don't like the things they're doing to her," she whispered. "I can't speak because we're being monitored."

There was something odd about this woman, and my father felt himself grow red in the face, embarrassed by the interaction. Still, he couldn't help but hear the woman out, especially since my own paranoid ravings seemed confirmed by her exhortations. Naturally, he worried about what occurred on the floor in his absence, although he knew deep down that the center was one of the best in the world and that these fears were likely imaginary.

"Here," she said, handing my dad a crumpled paper with illegible numbers scrawled across it. "Call me and I'll explain."

My dad politely put the number in his pocket, but he knew better than to call her. He pushed open the door to my new room, accidentally hitting the security guard whose chair had been propped up against it.

The new room was surprisingly peaceful, with a bank of windows looking out onto the East River and FDR Drive. Barges slipped silently by on their trips downriver. My father was pleased by the change, since he'd grown convinced that the AMU room with its monitors, nursing station, and the constant activity of the three other patients had heightened my anxiety.

When I finally awoke, I saw him and smiled. It was the first time that I had greeted him with warmth since that unspeakable night at his house, the evening before I was admitted. Heartened by my new attitude, he proposed a walk around the floor to keep me active.

Though I readily agreed to the walk, it wasn't easy to do. I maneuvered my body like an elderly person, stiffly easing myself toward the edge of the bed before dangling my feet over the side. My dad slid a fresh pair of nonskid, moss-colored socks over my feet and helped me off the bed. He noticed I had no electrodes on my head, but as it turned out this was just because I had removed them again during another overnight escape attempt, and the staff hadn't yet been able to replace them.

Even walking itself was no longer a simple task for me. My dad had always been a fast walker (when James and I were little, he often barreled ahead of us down crowded city streets), but now he was careful to stay by my side, guiding me as each leg jutted out and landed awkwardly, as if I was learning how to walk all over again. He couldn't help but drop the cheerful facade when he saw my slow movements. When we got back to my room, he suggested a motto to keep my mind on the silver lining.

"What is the slope of the line?" he asked.

I looked at him in silence.

"It's positive," he said with forced optimism, angling his arm upward to show a slope. "And what does positive mean?"

Another blank look.

"It means we make progress every day."

I was deteriorating physically, but at least my psychosis had receded, clearing the way for the doctors to finally schedule more tests. Whatever I suffered from seemed to ebb and flow, minute to minute, hour to hour. Still, the hospital staff jumped on this seeming progress and proceeded with a lumbar puncture, more commonly known as a spinal tap, which would give them access to the clear, saltwater-like cerebrospinal fluid that bathes the brain and spinal cord. The test had been too dangerous to conduct before because a lumbar puncture requires full cooperation from the patient to remain steadfastly still. Sudden movement can mean horrendous risks, including paralysis and even death.

Although my dad understood that the lumbar puncture was a necessary next step, the thought of the procedure still terrified him and my mom. When James was an infant, he had suffered from a dangerously high fever that had required a spinal tap to rule out meningitis, and my parents had never forgotten the baby's shrill, anguished screams.

The next day, March 27, was my fifth in the hospital but only the second time I had allowed my dad into my room. Most of the time I stared off into space, without any visible display of emotion, my psychosis now completely replaced by passivity. Still, these remote spells were sometimes punctuated by a few passionate pleas for help. In my few seemingly lucid moments (which are, like the rest of this time, still foggy or entirely blank in my own recollection), my dad felt as if some primal part of me was reaching out to him as I repeated over and over, "I'm dying in here. This place is killing me. Please let me leave." These invocations deeply pained my father. He desperately wanted me out of this soul-sucking situation, but he knew there was no other option than to stay.

Meanwhile, my mom, who had visited me that morning but had had to return to work downtown in the afternoon, worried from afar, checking in with my father periodically to get updates about the procedure. She hid her desperation from her coworkers, focusing instead on her heavy workload, but her thoughts kept circling around me. She tried unsuccessfully to concentrate on getting through the workday, telling herself over and over that she shouldn't feel guilty and that my father was looking after me.

Eventually, a young male orderly arrived to collect me for my spinal tap, calmly helping me from the bed into the wheelchair and motioning for my dad to follow. After they elbowed their way onto a cramped elevator, the orderly tried to make small talk.

"How are you two related?" he asked.

"I'm her father."

"Is she epileptic?"

My dad bristled. "No."

"Oh. I was just asking because I'm epileptic . . . ," the orderly said, trailing off apologetically.

He wheeled me from one elevator bank to another across the stadium-sized entranceway and finally into a holding pen that also housed five other gurneys, each with its own orderly and patient. My dad angled his body in front of my line of vision so that I would not be tempted to compare my own fate with those around me. *She is not one of these people,* he repeated endlessly to himself, until the nurse called me in alone. He knew I was just getting a spinal tap, but he couldn't help his mind wandering to more sinister scenarios. It was that kind of place.

CHAPTER 21

DEATH WITH INTERRUPTIONS

N early a week had gone by since I was admitted, but inside the hospital it was as if time didn't exist. Stephen likened the atmosphere to Atlantic City, with beeping blood pressure monitors instead of slot machines and sad, sick patients instead of sad, sick gamblers. Like a casino, there were no clocks or calendars. It was a stabilized, static environment; the only thing that punctuated the time was the endless activity of the nurses and doctors. From what my family could tell, I had developed an affection for two of the nurses: Edward and Adeline. Nurse Edward, a burly guy with a warm smile, was the only man on a floor of all female nurses, and because of this, he was often mistaken for a doctor. He took it in stride, maintaining an extraordinarily cheery disposition, and joked with me about the Yankees and the *New York Post,* his favorite newspaper. By contrast, Nurse Adeline, a middle-aged Filipino woman, was tigerishly efficient, a straight shooter who offered a healthy dose of discipline. Apparently she had a calming effect on me.

By now, my family had developed a routine. Now that I was again comfortable in his presence, my father would arrive in the morning, feed me a breakfast of yogurt and cappuccino, and play a few games of cards that I was often too disoriented to follow. Then he'd read aloud a book or magazine or just sit beside me quietly reading James Joyce's *Portrait of the Artist as a Young Man.* Every day he brought homemade gourmet foods like my favorite dessert, strawberry rhubarb pie, although I would often hand over my father's dishes to Stephen because I still was not eating regularly. My father had grown up watching his mother, an

Irish nurse, whip up elaborate dishes in between ER shifts, and, like her, he unwound when he cooked. Not only did it help me through those hospital days, but it also helped him concentrate on something besides the bleakness.

My mother arrived during her lunch hour and after work to check on me, always keeping that trusty list of questions by her side. Often she stared out at the view of the East River, watching the boats pass the Long Island City PEPSI COLA sign, wringing her hands, a nervous habit, and losing herself in the view. Most days, we'd watch the Yankees play, and she would give me a rundown of what was happening with our favorite players. But mostly she sat beside me, making sure I was comfortable and, above all else, that the best doctors were visiting regularly.

Stephen would arrive around 7:00 p.m. and stay until I fell asleep around midnight. The nursing staff okayed this, even though visiting hours had ended long before, because his calming influence meant that I would not try to escape. Every night Stephen and I watched a twenty-four-minute DVD of Ryan Adams at Austin City Limits, which was on a constant loop. He left it running when he went home, the alt-country songs "A Kiss Before I Go," "A Hard Way to Fall," and others playing like twangy lullabies over and over again until a night nurse, seeing that I'd fallen asleep, would turn the television off. Stephen thought the music might somehow help bring me back.

Instead, every time I watched this DVD, it was as if for the first time. My short-term memory had been obliterated, a problem usually rooted in the hippocampus, which is like a way station for new memories. The hippocampus briefly "stores" the patterns of neurons that make up a memory before passing them along to the parts of the brain responsible for preserving them long term. Memories are maintained by the areas of the brain responsible for the initial perception: a visual memory is saved by the visual cortex in the occipital lobe, an auditory memory by the auditory cortex of the temporal lobe, and so forth.

To understand how important the hippocampus is to the circuitry of the brain, all you have to do is consider what happens when it is removed, as in the famous case of the patient who became known to the medical world as H.M. In 1933, a bicycle struck seven-year-old Henry Gustav Molaison near his home in Hartford, Connecticut, knocking him out cold. After that fateful accident, H.M. experienced clusters of seizures that increased in intensity until, by his twenty-seventh birthday in 1953, his doctor had decided to remove the bit of brain tissue that seemed to be the focus of his seizures: the hippocampus. When H.M. recovered from the surgery, the seizures were gone, but too went his ability to make memories. The doctors noticed that his old memories were intact up to two years before the surgery, but he could no longer retain new ones. Any new information stayed with him for a mere twenty seconds before it vanished. H.M. lived into his eighties, but always thought of himself as a young man in his mid-twenties, the age he was before his surgery.

His uniquely terrifying situation made him one of the most famous medical studies in history, helping researchers to confirm the existence of anterograde amnesia, or the inability to create new memories. (The movie *Memento* is modeled after H.M.) His case also established the existence of two different types of memory: declarative (places, names, object, facts, and events) and procedural (those learned as a habit, like tying shoes or riding a bike). Although H.M. could not make any new declarative memories, he retained his procedural memory, which he could unconsciously strengthen with practice.

More recently, an orchestra conductor named Clive Wearing contracted a devastating form of herpes simplex encephalitis that ravaged his brain, destroying his hippocampus. Like H.M., Wearing could not retain any new declarative memories, meaning that his world was constantly new to him. He couldn't recognize his children, and whenever he saw his wife, to whom he had been married for years, he felt as if he was falling in love for the first time. His wife, Deborah, wrote a book about his case, aptly titled *Forever Today*. In it she wrote: "Clive was under the constant impression that he had just emerged from unconsciousness because he had no evidence in his own mind of ever being awake before." A prolific writer himself, Wearing kept lengthy diaries. But instead of filling them with insight or humor, he was constantly writing the following:

8:31 AM: Now I am really, completely awake.

9:06 AM: Now I am perfectly, overwhelmingly awake.

9:34 AM: Now I am superlatively, actually awake.

Deborah quotes her husband: "I haven't heard anything, seen anything, touched anything, smelled anything. It's like being dead."

Although my case luckily was not yet as severe as these, I too had lost key parts of my brain function. Still, certain little things brought me joy: I looked forward to the slow, rickety walks that allowed me to skip the daily shots required to prevent blood clots in bedridden patients. Beyond that, I had two other obsessions, apples and cleanliness. Whenever anybody asked me what I wanted, my answer was always the same: "Apples." I expressed a constant desire for them, so everyone who visited brought apples: green ones, red ones, tart ones, sweet ones. I devoured them all. I don't know what prompted this fixation; perhaps some metaphorical urge to "have an apple a day, and keep the doctor away." Or maybe the urge was more basic: apples contain flavonoids, which are known to have anti-inflammatory and antioxidant effects on the body. Was my body communicating something that my mind—and my doctors—didn't yet understand?

I also insisted on having my clothes changed and cleaned every day. My mother believed this was a subconscious yearning to rid my body of the sickness, whatever it was. I begged the staff to shower me, even though my hair had to remain matted to my skull because of the constant presence of the EEG wires. Two Jamaican nursing assistants would clean me with warm wet towels, dress me, and coo over me, calling me "my baby." I relaxed in their care. Watching my contentment during these washing sessions, my father wondered if their accents were transporting me back to my infancy, when Sybil had cared for me like a second mother.

That first Saturday, my parents finally allowed a new visitor, my cousin Hannah. Though she was shocked by what she saw when she arrived, Hannah walked in the room and sat down next to me as if she had done this every day. There in the room with my mom and Stephen, she seemed immediately at home, quiet, unassuming, and supportive.

"Susannah, these are from your birthday. We didn't get to see you," she said brightly, handing me a wrapped present. I stared blankly back at her with a frozen smile. Hannah and I had made plans in February to celebrate my belated birthday, but I had canceled because of the "mono" that I believed I had contracted.

"Thank you," I said. Hannah watched hesitantly as I clawed weakly at the present with half-closed fists. I no longer had the dexterity to even open the wrapping paper. My physical slowness and awkward speech pattern reminded Hannah of a Parkinson's patient. Gently she took the package from me and opened it.

"It's *Death with Interruptions*," she said. "You liked *All the Names*, so my mom and I thought you'd like this one, too." In college I had read José Saramago's *All the Names* and spent many nights talking to Hannah's mother about it. But now I just glanced helplessly at the author's name and said, "Never read that." Hannah agreed sweetly and changed the subject.

"She's really tired," my mother apologized. "It's hard for her to concentrate."

EEG video, March 30, 6:50 a.m., 6 minutes

The scene opens onto an empty bed. My mother, dressed in a Max Mara suit for work, sits nearby, looking pensively out the window. There are flowers and magazines by the bed. The TV is on, and the show *Everybody Loves Raymond* plays softly.

I enter from offscreen and crawl onto the bed. I do not have my cap on, and my hair is matted down, revealing a strip of wires that fall down my back like a mane. I pull the sheets up to my neck. My mother rubs my thigh and tucks me into the blanket. I remove the blanket and get up, repeatedly touching the wires on my head.

End of video.

CHAPTER 22
A BEAUTIFUL MESS

Troubling new symptoms cropped up in the beginning of the second week. My mother had arrived midmorning to find that my slurring of words had worsened so considerably that it was as if my tongue was five sizes too big for my mouth. This scared her more than the hallucinations, the paranoia, and the escape attempts: this was measurable, consistent change, but in decidedly the wrong direction. My tongue twisted when I spoke; I drooled and, when I was tired, let my tongue hang out of the side of my mouth like an overheated dog; I spoke in garbled sentences; I coughed when I drank liquids, which required that I drink water out of a cup that dispensed only a tablespoon of liquid at a time; I also stopped speaking in full sentences, moving from unintelligible ramblings to monosyllables and sometimes just grunts. "Can you repeat after me?" Dr. Russo, the neurologist, asked. "Ca, ca, ca."

But the hard sounds of the c's coming from my mouth were so softened that the consonant became unrecognizable, more like "dtha, dtha, dtha."

"Would you please puff out your cheeks, like this?" Dr. Russo asked, blowing into her closed mouth, extending her cheeks. I pursed my lips and mimed the doctor, but the air would not fill my cheeks. I just exhaled.

"Will you point your tongue out all the way at me?"

My tongue would extend only about half the length of a normal person's, and even so, it quivered as if strained by the action.

Later that day, Dr. Arslan confirmed Dr. Russo's new findings, noting my slurred speech in his progress report. I was also making constant chewing motions, not unlike the lip licking in Summit the week before. And now I was making weird grimaces too. My arms kept stiffening out in front of me, as if I was reaching for something that wasn't there. The team suspected that these behaviors, combined with the high blood pressure and increased heart rate, pointed to a problem in my brain stem or limbic system.

At the top of the spinal cord and at the underside of the brain is the brain stem, one of the more primitive parts of the brain, which helps oversee basic life-or-death functions. A thumb-sized cluster of cells in the brain stem called the medulla manages blood pressure, heart rate, and breathing. A bulging area nearby, the pons, plays an important role in the control of facial expressions, so it made sense that my symptoms might be coming from this area.

Still, it's hard to lay blame. Many areas of the brain are also involved with these kinds of intrinsic functions. Other possible culprits are the insular cortex, located between the frontal and temporal lobes, which is involved with emotion and maintenance of the body's internal environment; or they could be caused by parts of the limbic system, such as the amygdala and the cingulate gyrus, which are involved with respiratory control.

To return to the analogy of the Christmas lights, even if just one area goes out, many different connections may be altered. It's often difficult to locate one area and make a causal connection to basic functions or behavior. Just like everything else in the brain, it's complicated. Or, as author William F. Allman put it in *Apprentices of Wonder: Inside the Neural Network Revolution*, "The brain is a monstrous, beautiful mess."

Dr. Siegel (my mom's beloved "Bugsy") arrived with news shortly after Dr. Arslan had left. "All right, we have something," he said, speaking rapidly.

"Something?" my mother asked.

"Her spinal tap showed a slightly elevated level of white blood cells. This is typically a sign that there is some kind of infection or inflammation," he said. There were twenty white blood cells in my spinal fluid in about a microliter of fluid; in a healthy person's spinal fluid, there should be only zero to five. It was enough for the doctors to wonder, but there were various theories as to why they were there. One of the possible explanations was that they'd been caused by the trauma of the spinal tap itself. Still, it was an indication that something was awry.

"We don't know what it means yet," Dr. Siegel said. "We've got dozens of tests going. We'll figure it out. I promise you we will figure it out."

My mother smiled for the first time in weeks. It was a strange relief for her to finally have confirmation that something physical, as opposed to emotional, was happening to me. She desperately wanted something—anything that she could wrap her mind around. And although this white blood cell clue was vague, it was nonetheless a clue. She went home and spent the rest of the evening on Google, researching what this news could mean. The possibilities were frightening: meningitis, tumor, stroke, multiple sclerosis. Eventually a phone call interrupted her research trance. My voice on the other end sounded like a developmentally delayed child.

"I peed."

"What happened?"

"I peed. They're yelling."

"Who's yelling at you?" She could hear voices in the background.

"Nurses. I peed. I didn't mean to."

"Susannah. They're not mad at you. I promise. It's their job to clean it up. They know you didn't do it on purpose."

"They're yelling at me."

"I promise you it's not a big deal. It happens. They shouldn't yell. It was a mistake." She couldn't tell what was real and what had been engineered by my tortured mind. Allen agreed that it was likely the latter; either way, they never heard anything more about the incident.

. . .

Because I was still paranoid about work and seemed ashamed about my condition, my parents kept my hospital stay a secret from almost everyone, even my brother. But on Tuesday, March 31, as the first week folded into a second, my parents allowed my first nonfamily friend, Katie, to come visit me. Katie and I had met in college and bonded over a shared love for Loretta Lynn, soul music, vintage clothes, and stiff St. Louis cocktails. Katie was vibrant, a bit goofy, and a great partner in crime. Not knowing what to bring, she purchased a stuffed rat (Katie in a nutshell: a rat instead of a teddy bear), a DVD of gangster rap videos, and a subtitled French film, not realizing that I could no longer read.

Katie now worked as a teacher in Queens and had coached many children with serious social issues and learning difficulties, but she was unprepared for what she found on the other side of the hospital door. This new me was physically different: skinny and pale, cheeks sunken in, and thighs whittled down to toothpicks. My eyes were glazed over. Trying to break the ice, Katie gossiped about people we had gone to college with, knowing that her role was to distract me from the serious matters around me. But it was hard to maintain a conversation because I operated on a delay, responding to basic questions several seconds after they were posed. And then there was the problem of my speech. I had been a professional conversationalist, normally the kind of person who could make small talk with a brick wall, but this new me struggled with even the simplest statements. Most of the time Katie couldn't even make out what I was saying.

"Let's go for a walk," Katie suggested, joking, "Don't forget your Dora the Explorer backpack." It took me several moments to realize that Katie was referring to the little pink bag that carried my EEG wires, but eventually I laughed. We shuffled slowly to the waiting area and sat on two chairs facing away from the windows. Katie noticed how baggy my black leggings were.

"You're so skinny, Susannah!"

I looked down at my legs for a moment, like I was discovering a new part of my body. I laughed and said: "Theeeeeessssseearrrrre my

legggggggggggggings! My legggggggggggings! My leggggggggggggings!"
and got out of my seat to perform an awkward Irish jig. Weird, yes,
but I was dancing, so Katie took that as a good sign.

After Katie's visit, the next friends to come were Angela and Julie
from work. Angela hadn't seen me since the emotional evening at
the Marriott Hotel when I couldn't stop crying. Since then I had
called her a few times in the middle of the night, breathing heavily into the phone but saying nothing. Julie had spoken to me
once since the day that she suggested that I was bipolar, when she
phoned me in the hospital. The only thing I could offer was, "I
had pie for breakfast."

Today, when I knew they were coming, I'd asked for one thing:
a cheeseburger. As they carried the burgers and fries up in the elevator, neither one was sure what to expect.

They walked into the hospital room and found my cousin
Hannah seated beside me, keeping me company. I was clearly
happy to see them. I gave them a fixed but wide, toothy smile as
they tried to ignore the shock of seeing me with my white hat and
those multicolored wires. Angela handed me a cheeseburger, but I
put it on the bedside table, untouched, and later gave it to Stephen
when he arrived that night. Julie, never one to be shy, immediately
jumped into bed next to me. She dug her cell phone out of her bag
and scrolled through her pictures until she found the right one.

"Do you want to see a picture?" she asked, and all four girls
hovered around the phone. "It's my poop!"

Everyone but me gasped.

"They wouldn't let me leave the hospital after Teddy was born
until I took one. I was so proud that I took a picture." Julie had
given birth to her son about a month earlier. Angela and Hannah
started laughing hysterically as I grabbed the cell phone, peered
in close, and, several seconds later, broke out into hysterical, near
sobbing laughs. The three others looked at each other and lost

it again. I seemed happy and more with it during these visits. As Stephen had noticed, I seemed to be able to somehow pull myself together when I had visitors, but it would often leave me depleted and unable to communicate for hours afterward, as if I had devoted all my energy to acting normal.

Angela, ever the reporter, immediately began asking questions. "Susannah, what's going on here?"

"I . . . don't . . . remember," I stuttered. A little while later I interrupted a separate conversation, my voice suddenly clearer but still just as slow: "What are people saying about me?"

"Don't worry about it. No one is saying anything about it. They're all just concerned," Angela replied.

"No, tell me. I want to know."

"Nothing bad, Susannah. Nothing bad. I promise."

"I know that Gawker has been saying bad things about me," I insisted, referring to the gossip blog.

Julie and Angela threw each other a strange look. "What do you mean?"

"Gawker. It's saying bad things about me. They put my name in the headline of a piece," I said and sat up in bed, deadly serious. "Should I call them?"

Angela shook her head. "Um, no. That's probably not a good idea. Why don't you write an e-mail when you're feeling better?"

After about an hour, Angela and Julie said their good-byes and walked down the hallway to the elevators. They pushed the button, still in silence, and waited. When they got in, Julie said quietly, "Do you think she's ever going to be the same?"

It was a fair question. The person whom Angela and Julie had just visited was not the one they had been friends with for so many years.

But still, there was something of me that remained. Though I could no longer concentrate enough to read, I still had some ability to write, so my father gave me a lined notebook to record how I felt, to help me communicate with visitors and help them better understand what was going on.

~~Headaches~~
Headaches
Problems ~~remembey~~ ~~how to~~ ~~co~~ret

~~Brab~~
My problems &
Brain Remembery how to to spell things
Recogniy tnp tnp
Writy thing down
recaly words
concentrehnher
dizziness

In addition to tracking my difficulties in the notebook, I became temporarily obsessed with thanking the various people who had sent me flowers. All sorts of arrangements had been arriving in my room: white daffodils, yellow tulips, pink roses, orange sunflowers, and pink and white lilies (my favorite). I begged my father to help make a list of the people to send thank-you notes once I felt better. When I got too tired to continue writing, my father wrote out some of the names and short thank-you notes for me. But I never got the opportunity to send them out. Because things would get worse before they would get better.

The blood test had come back from the Centers for Disease Control and the New York State labs: everything was negative. The doctors now had a long list of the things I did not have. The infectious disease panel included:

- Lyme disease, often caused by tick bites

- Toxoplasmosis, a parasitic disease usually carried by cats

- Cryptococcus, a type of fungus that can cause meningitis

- Tuberculosis, which affects the lungs

- Lymphoreticulosis, or "cat scratch fever"

The autoimmune panel of tests, which tests for some but not all of the 100 plus autoimmune diseases, also came back negative, including:

- Sjögren's syndrome, which affects the glands that produce tears and saliva

- Multiple sclerosis, which harms the fatty layer of myelin that sheaths neurons

- Lupus, a connective tissue disease

- Scleroderma, a disease of the skin

Nada. Nothing had come back abnormal. Even the various MRIs and CT scans were clean. If the labs were to be believed, I was 100 percent healthy. My parents could sense that the doctors were starting to despair that they would never figure it out. And if there wasn't a physical problem to cure, everyone understood—though no one would admit—that I would be on my way out to a far worse place. At this point, my family needed someone who would believe in me no matter what. This was the only time in my mother's long experience with doctors that she had hoped for positive test results. At least then we would have an answer.

My mom had started to look forward every day to seeing the grandfatherly Dr. "Bugsy"; his perpetual good cheer and kind words had become one of the only bright spots in these darkening days. When he didn't arrive on the afternoon that the test results came back, she worried, and wandered the hallway looking for him. She spied his white lab coat as he left one of the other rooms down the hall.

"Oh, Dr. Siegel," she said, her voice rising on the end of his name. He turned around swiftly without smiling, evidently in a hurry. "What's going on with Susannah? Anything new?"

He stared back without his familiar warmth and optimism. "I'm not on the case anymore," he said flatly and turned to leave.

"What, what?" she stammered, her lower lip quivering. "What do we do?"

"I don't know what to say. It's no longer my case," he replied. He turned and walked briskly away. She suddenly felt very alone. There had been many low points throughout my illness, but this rebuff was the lowest. This doctor, one of the best in the country, had now, it seemed, given up on me.

She took another deep breath, straightened out her blazer, and headed back into my room. She felt foolish for believing that I had been anything but a patient—one in a series of numbers—to him. She could hardly stand to look at Dr. Russo when she came in later that afternoon. Now she was our only hope—that is, until Dr. Russo, as she was finishing up the examination, turned to my mother and said, "Dr. Najjar and I feel that a second spinal tap is now necessary."

My deteriorating condition made the idea of another spinal tap, once so frightening, now seem insignificant. But my mother clung to the mention of a new doctor. "Who is Dr. Najjar?"

"He's working on your daughter's case. He's a brilliant doctor," Dr. Russo said.

Dr. Souhel Najjar had joined my team after a call from Dr. Siegel. His skill in solving a few mystery cases had earned him a reputation as the man to go to when nothing made sense. And now Dr. Bugsy was offering up his most perplexing case to him.

"I'm at a loss," Dr. Siegel confided to Dr. Najjar. "I need your help on this case." He listed all the issues and conflicting diagnoses. The psychiatrists suspected that my behavior stemmed from a mental illness; the elevated white blood cell count pointed to infection; all the other tests were coming back negative. Dr. Najjar's first guess was that I had to be suffering from some sort of viral encephalitis, an inflammation most likely caused by the herpes virus. He didn't buy the schizoaffective theory and instead suggested that they administer an infusion of IV acyclovir, an antiviral drug.

But then the virus panel came back negative. I did not have HIV or herpes simplex virus 1 or 2 and did not test positive for herpes encephalitis, so he stopped the antiviral infusions. The other possibility was that it was some sort of autoimmune response, which he could treat with an experimental immunotherapy that he had tried successfully on another patient with brain inflammation; the treatment included steroids, intravenous immunoglobulin (IVIG), and plasma exchange.

"I think we should do IVIG treatment immediately," Dr. Najjar said after looking over my negative virus panel.

CHAPTER 24
IVIG

On April 2, the nurses started my first round of five intravenous immunoglobulin (IVIG) infusions. The clear IV bags hung on a metal pole above my head, their liquid trickling down into my vein. Each of those ordinary-looking bags contained the healthy antibodies of over a thousand blood donors and cost upwards of $20,000 per infusion. One thousand tourniquets, one thousand nurses, one thousand veins, one thousand blood-sugar regulating cookies, all just to help one patient.

IVIG is made up of serum antibodies called immunoglobulin G, or IgG, which are the most common type of antibody found in the human body. IVIG is approved by the U.S. Food and Drug Administration to treat problems relating to transplants, leukemia, and pediatric HIV, among other conditions; its off-label uses have often been considered "experimental" and denied by insurance companies.

Antibodies are created by the body's immune system to counteract an unwanted, external element, such as when a pathogen of some sort—a virus, bacterium, fungus, or other foreign substance—enters the body. This sets off a series of reactions beginning with the body's basic alarm system, the innate response, which is a one-size-fits-all process designed to get rid of unwanted visitors quickly. If the innate system can't eradicate the pathogen, the next defense stage is the "adaptive response," which tailors itself to the specific intruder, using an arsenal of white blood cells and antibodies. This takes much longer to mobilize than the innate response, ten days versus the innate system's minutes or hours. Usually the collateral damage of these internal battles results in familiar flulike symptoms such as headache, fever, muscle ache, nausea, and enlarged lymph nodes.

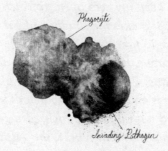

An immune cell, called a phagocyte, "eating" a pathogen.

One type of white blood cell, the B-cell, also can morph into plasma cells that create antibodies. Under normal conditions, each antibody fits exactly to only one pathogen, like Cinderella's glass slipper, with the purpose of blocking the spread of infection by either disabling that specific kind of pathogen or flagging it for destruction. But autoantibodies, which everyone has in healthy doses, can sometimes transform into the most malicious type of biological shadowboxer, if they begin to attach to and destroy the healthy host tissue, like the brain. An IVIG infusion introduces fresh, healthy antibodies to fuse with those "bad" rogue autoantibodies created by a sick person's immune system, helping to neutralize them and rendering the autoantibodies harmless.

Beep, beep, beep. It's dark. There's the beeping of a massive machine to my right. There's a wire hooking me up to heaving bags of white liquid. I put Stephen's headphones on and close my eyes. I am far, far away from here. I am myself again.

"This next song is to my friend Leah who couldn't be here tonight . . ."

The hum of the guitar. The soft tap on the drums. The swell of the music. It's Halloween night at Harlem's Apollo Theater. I'm at a Ryan Adams concert. I can see him onstage, strumming on his guitar, but I can't keep my eyes open to watch the scene. I feel a touch on my skin. It makes me shudder. I hear a voice.

"SuSHana, time to take vitals."

The concert disappears, dissolving into the dark hospital room, the nurse next to me. I'm back, back in the place where there is no night and there is no day. It's this woman's fault I'm back here. I'm suddenly filled with blinding, focused rage. I wind my right arm back and punch her in the chest. She gasps.

The next morning, my mother took her usual place beside me in a chair by the window when her phone rang. It was James. My parents had been keeping him uninformed about the severity of my illness, not wanting to worry him and disrupt his studies. He and I had always been close, despite the five-year age difference, and our parents knew he would drop everything and come home if he discovered how bad off I was. But today, for the first time, she decided to hand off the phone to me.

"James . . . James . . . James," I said, hearing my brother's voice on the other line. "James . . . James . . . James."

In his dorm room in Pittsburgh, James choked back tears. I sounded so different, so unlike his big sister. He insisted, "I'm going to come home soon. And you're going to get better."

·······

The following day, while I was on my second course of IVIG treatment, Dr. Arslan, the psychopharmacologist, came by on rounds and noticed that my speech problems had worsened. He wrote the following in his progress note:

Some sleep problems overnight and increased speech latency, the latter a concern because it may be an initial catatonic sign. Seroquel less effectve for sleep last night than previously.

It was the first time that anyone had mentioned the term *catatonia*, a stage defined by absence, by inability, by nonbehaviors. The mnemonic that doctors use to diagnose catatonia is WIRED 'N MIRED:

- Waxy flexibility/catalepsy (muscular rigidity and fixedness of posture)

- Immobility/stupor

- Refusal to eat or drink

- Excitement

- Deadpan staring

- Negativism/negative symptoms

- Mutism

- Impulsivity

- Rigidity

- Echolalia (automatic repetition of words or statements said by another person)

- Direct observation

Catatonia comes from the misfiring of neurons. That "muscular rigidity," also called posturing, occurs when the chemical link is severed between the patient's awareness of her body and the feeling of comfort and appropriateness of movement. In other words, a catatonic patient cannot sense his or her body in space, and therefore cannot appropriately adjust. The result is that a person sits very still in awkward, atypical, unnatural poses. Catatonia is more akin to the results of a botched lobotomy than a persistent vegetative state because the person is technically still active. There are behaviors of a sort, as bizarre, nonresponsive, and inappropriate as they may be.

Meanwhile, a comment that the nurse had made the night before was haunting Stephen. She was a young Asian immigrant who had just begun working at New York University. While examining me, she said offhandedly, "Has she always been so slow?"

Stephen shook his head violently, struggling to control his temper. *How dare she say something like that. Susannah is not, and never was, slow.*

The next morning, Stephen ran into my father in the hallway. At first, they spoke about superficial things—the cold weather, how Stephen's work was, and so forth. But the conversation quickly turned to me.

"She's still in there," Stephen said. "I can see her. She's still there. I know it."

"I agree. And that's who we're fighting for. None of the doctors and nurses see it, but we do," my dad said. "And we have to remain strong for her."

"Agreed." The two men shook hands. My dad wrote about his new impression of Stephen in his journal: "The one friend who did come everyday was Stephen. He was terrific. I wasn't that sold on him when I first met him, but he grew in my respect and regard with every day that passed."

CHAPTER 25

BLUE DEVIL FIT

They did the second lumbar puncture on April 9. I had been in the hospital for eighteen days, and not only wasn't I any closer to a cure, but my condition seemed to be heading steadily downhill. For one, Stephen had noticed that my constant chewing motions, my bride-of-Frankenstein arm movements, and my staring episodes had become more frequent.

EEG video, April 8, 10:30 p.m., 11 minutes

The TV blares a Discovery channel reality show.

Stephen sits beside me watching the show with his hand on my thigh as I sleep on my side, facing him. Stephen turns to me. Suddenly I sit up and start to inhale rapidly without exhaling. He strokes my hair. My arms rise straight out in front of me as Stephen snatches up the nurse's alarm button. He stands over me, watching in horror as I slowly bend my hands to my face. I do this so leadenly that it looks like stop-motion animation. A nurse arrives. She speaks with Stephen, but the blaring television program masks their conversation. I don't say a word. Stephen tries to explain what happened, miming choking to show her that I had stopped breathing. I extend my arms straight out again while he speaks, but my hands are bent downward at the wrists like those of a *T. rex.* Stephen gently places them back by my sides and rubs my shoulders, but my hands return to the extended position with that forty-five-degree angle at the wrist, as if held up by strings. I begin to move them in rapid, repetitive motions, up and down, up and down. Then I put my hands back to my face and lie down stiffly until an on-call neurologist arrives.

Stephen again tries to show the doctor what happened, clench-ing his arms and gritting his teeth. Stressed and terrified, he starts to cry. I toss a nearby teddy bear to the floor and bat the air awk-wardly like I'm fending off a ghost—but with my arms so rigid I look like a Barbie doll going into battle. The doctor asks me a few questions that are too muffled to make out, but I do not answer, just stare off. I lie back down.

I then sit up again and try to get out of bed, but the guardrail stops me. The doctor lowers the guardrail and hands me a pail, pos-sibly because she believes I'm nauseous. I sway back and forth. I lie back down with the pail between my legs. The doctor takes it from me and places it by my head.

End of video.

During moments like these, Stephen couldn't will the night of the initial seizure on March 13 out of his mind. "What do you think that was?" Stephen asked Nurse Adeline later that night.

"Maybe she was just trying to get your attention?" South-erners called attention-seeking attacks "blue devil fits," a vivid description of temper tantrums or anxiety attacks exhibited by young women. "Maybe it was some sort of an anxiety attack?"

Stephen didn't buy this explanation. The next night, the same thing happened.

"I . . . don't . . . feel . . . gooooood," I said, angling my legs off the bed. Stephen followed my lead and lowered the guardrail and guided me out of bed and onto the floor. I began heaving for air again and crying. Stephen pushed the call button.

"My . . . heart . . . hurtsssssssss . . . ," I said, holding my chest and squirming on the cold hospital floor. "I . . . can't . . . breeee-athe."

A nurse came rushing in. She took my vital signs and noted slightly increased blood pressure of 155/97. She hooked me up to a two-liter oxygen machine that can help with cardiac issues and convulsions. Soon after, I fell asleep. Variations on the same scene would happen over and over almost every night when Stephen was visiting. They rarely happened with anyone else. No one ever provided an explanation.

—◆—

My whole family was growing increasingly wayworn as time went on and no one seemed to have an answer. All the tests continued to come back negative, the immunoglobulin treatments didn't seem to be the magic elixir that everyone had hoped they would be, and no one had been able to figure out what the high white blood cell count might be suggesting. Worse, Dr. Bugsy was now off the case, and this Dr. Najjar, whom everyone spoke so highly of, still hadn't made an appearance. What would stop the others from giving up too and condemning me to a mental institution or a nursing home? Quietly, secretly, despite all their steadfast optimism, my family began to worry that if things continued to go downhill, they really might lose me forever.

The next day, the results from the spinal tap came back. Dr. Russo delivered the news, which was alarming but at least meant they were nearing an answer: my cerebrospinal fluid had eighty white blood cells in about a microliter of cerebrospinal fluid, up from twenty the week before. This meant that my brain was almost certainly inflamed; now they just had to figure out what was causing it. When I arrived on the floor, the chief complaint was seizures; then it was changed to psychosis; now Russo wrote down "encephalitis of an unknown origin." Encephalitis, one neurologist would eventually explain, colloquially meant "bad brain," or the inflammation of the brain due to a host of causes.

Since my mom hadn't been there for Dr. Russo's visit, my dad jotted the news down in their shared logbook:

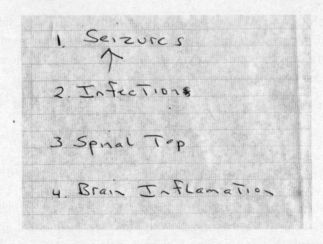

He tried to communicate the good news to me, but I couldn't follow. "Why don't you copy what I've written, and write a few extra things as I tell you," he said.

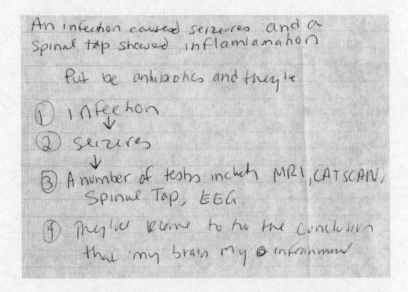

We imagined that when people came to visit, I could hand over this paper, hoping it would tell the whole story. The plan didn't last long: By the time Hannah arrived that same day, I could not find the notebook. It had been lost among the flowers and magazines that packed the hospital room. "I have, I have . . ." I struggled to explain. Hannah slid into bed beside me and laced her arms around my neck.

"I have, I have, I have . . ." I said.

"It's okay, Susannah, just drop it. You're tired," my mother interrupted.

"No. I want to," I stammered. My whole body tensed. "I . . . want . . . to . . . speak!"

"You're tired, sweetie. You should rest," my mom said.

I exhaled angrily. My mom understood that I was deeply frustrated by my inabilities and by being babied. Hannah sensed my irritation and distracted me with a month's worth of *US Weekly* magazines and the copy of *Catcher in the Rye* that I had begged her for. Because I could no longer read on my own, Hannah read to me until I closed my eyes to sleep. Suddenly, though, I looked up at her.

"Tlantyoiforslen," I said. "Tlantyoiforslen! Tlantyoiforslen!" I began repeating over and over, my face reddening.

"You're welcome," Hannah said, uncertainly.

I shook my head violently. "No, no, no!"

"Tlantyoiforslen!!!" I yelled. Hannah bent down closer to my face, but proximity only made me more unintelligible. I began pointing emphatically toward the door.

"Slefeen, sleefen!"

Finally, Hannah understood. She called Stephen in, and when I saw him, I instantly calmed.

The next day, taking a cue from my high white blood cell count, the doctors began looking for the source of my infection. A new set of blood tests was pending, so Nurse Edward came to draw blood. Stephen sat beside me, impressed by my demeanor today.

Though I was far from my old self, bits of my old humor seemed to have resurfaced. I smiled more, and appeared more engaged with the Yankees game, even commenting that I loved pitcher Andy Pettitte.

"How's the game?" Nurse Edward asked. "Are the Mets winning?" He made a joke. I held out my arm. I had done this so many times that it was all rote now. Edward put on his gloves; placed a tourniquet around my right forearm; prepped the vein, tapping it with his fingers; and bent down to insert the needle. But as the needle punctured my skin, I jumped up violently and in one quick motion slapped the needle out of his hand, sending blood spurting out of my vein. I smiled, looking down in mock sheepishness, as if to say, sarcastically, "Oops, what have I done?" It was obvious to Stephen that I meant, "Fuck off." Sometimes when I seemed to be doing better, the original psychosis would return. This frightened everyone.

"Susannah, please don't do that. You can really get hurt and maybe hurt me. But it's going to hurt you a lot more," Edward said, keeping his voice under control. He prepared the needle again and raised it over my outstretched arm.

"Okay," I said mildly. He inserted the needle, withdrew a few tubes of blood, and walked out of the room.

"**W**aher," I moaned, pointing to a pink pitcher on my bedside table. It was the day we were finally expecting Dr. Najjar to make an appearance. I was drooling and smacking my lips, a habit that now went on constantly, even while I slept. My dad put down his playing cards, picked up the pitcher, and walked out to the hallway to refill it. He returned to find me staring straight ahead. It seemed as if I were sleeping with my eyes open, my tongue hanging out of my mouth. By this point, he was so used to these scenes he took it all in stride. Instead of waking me, he silently read *A Portrait of the Artist as a Young Man* until my mother arrived.

"Hello," my mother said cheerily, entering the room. She propped her leather bag on the chair by the bed and kissed me. "I'm so excited to finally meet the mysterious Dr. Najjar today. What do you think he'll be like?" she continued brightly, enthusiasm radiating from her almond-shaped eyes. "He should be here any moment."

Enthusiasm was hard for my dad this morning. "I don't know, Rhona," he said. "We don't know anything yet."

She shrugged him off and grabbed a tissue to wipe the drool pooling on the side of my face.

"Hello, hello!" A few minutes later, Dr. Najjar strode into my private room, 1276, his voice booming. He had a measured gait and a slight slope to his back that made his head fall a few inches in front of his body, most likely due to the hours he spent hunched over a microscope. His thick mustache was worn at the tips from his habit of twisting and pulling at it when he was deep in thought.

He extended his hand to my mother, who, in her eagerness, held it firmly a bit longer than normal. Then he introduced himself to my father, who rose to greet him from the chair by my bed.

"Let's go through her medical history with you before I begin," he said. His Syrian accent hopped rhythmically, sticking on and accentuating the hard consonants, often turning t's into d's. When he got excited, he dropped prepositions and combined words, as if his speech could not keep up with his thoughts. Dr. Najjar always stressed the importance of getting a full health history from his patients. ("You have to look backward to see the future," he often said to his residents.) As my parents spoke, he took note of symptoms—headaches, bedbug scare, flulike symptoms, numbness, and the increased heart rate—that the other doctors had not explored, at least not in one full picture. He jotted these all down as key findings. And then he did something none of the other doctors had done: Dr. Najjar redirected his attention and spoke directly to me, as if I was his friend instead of his patient.

One of the remarkable things about Dr. Najjar was his very personal, heartfelt bedside manner. He had an intense sympathy for the weak and powerless, which, as he told me later, came from his own experiences as a little boy growing up in Damascus, Syria. He had done poorly in school, and his parents and teachers had considered him lazy. When he was ten, after he failed test after test in his private Catholic school, his principal had told his parents that he was beyond help: "Education is not for everyone. Maybe it would be best for him to learn a trade." Angry as he was, his father didn't want to stop his schooling—education was far too important—so although he didn't have high hopes, he put his son in public school instead.

During his first year at public school, one teacher took a special interest in the boy and often made a point to praise him for his work, slowly raising his confidence. By the end of that year, he came home with a glowing, straight A report card. His father was apoplectic.

"You cheated," Salim said, raising his hand to punish his son. The next morning, his parents confronted the teacher. "My son doesn't get these types of grades. He must be cheating."

"No, he's not cheating. I can assure you of that."

"Then what kind of school are you running here, where a boy like Souhel can get these kinds of grades?"

The teacher paused before speaking again. "Did you ever think that you might actually have a smart son? I think you need to believe in him."

Dr. Najjar would eventually graduate at the top of his class in medical school and immigrate to the United States, where he not only became an esteemed neurologist but also an epileptologist and neuropathologist. His own story carried with it a moral that applied to all of his patients: he was determined never to give up on any of them.

Now, in my hospital room, he crouched down beside me and said, "I will do my best to help you. I will not hurt you." I didn't say anything, looking emotionless. "Okay, let's begin. What is your name?"

A considerable pause. "Su . . . sa . . . nnn . . . aaah."

"What is the year?"

Pause. "2009." He wrote down "monosyllabic."

"What is the month?"

Pause. "Appril. Appril." I struggled here. He wrote "indifferent," meaning apathetic.

"What is the date?"

I looked forward, showing no emotion, saying nothing, not blinking. He wrote down "paucity of eye blinking." I didn't have an answer for him on this one.

"Who is the president?"

Pause. I raised my hand rigidly in front of me. He wrote "stiff-bodied" on his chart. "Wha?" No emotions. Nothing.

"Who is the president?" He noted "lack of attention span."

"O, Obama." He wrote, "low tone, monotonous with a substantial lisp." I was not able to control the movements of my tongue. He removed a few tools from his white lab coat. Using a reflex hammer, he tapped on my kneecaps, which did not jerk forward the way they should. He shined a light into my eyes, noting that my pupils were not properly constricting.

"Okay, now, touch your nose with this hand," he said, touching my right arm. Stiffly and robotically, I raised my arm and in several slow-moving motions, reached my hand to my face, narrowly missing my nose. *Hellishly catatonic,* he thought.

"Okay," he said, testing my ability to do a two-step command. "Touch your left ear with your left hand." He grazed my left arm to indicate right from left, doubting I could figure it out myself. I didn't move or react; instead, I just sighed. He told me to forget about this step and moved on to another. "I'd like you to get out of bed and walk for me." I dangled my feet over the edge and slid haltingly onto the floor. He took my arm and helped me stand. "Will you walk a straight line, one foot after the other?" he asked.

Taking a minute to think it through, I began walking in short spurts but with delays between steps. I angled toward my left side—Najjar noticed I was showing signs of ataxia, a lack of coordinated movement. I walked and talked like many of his late-stage Alzheimer's patients, who have lost their capacities to speak and appropriately interact with their environments, save for short bursts of uncontrolled, abnormal movements. They do not smile, hardly blink, and remain unnaturally rigid, with one foot firmly planted in another world. And then he had an idea: the clock test. Although developed in the mid-1950s, the clock test had been entered into the American Psychiatric Association's *Diagnostic and Statistical Manual of Mental Disorders* only in 1987 and is used to diagnose problem areas of the brain in Alzheimer's, stroke, and dementia patients.

Dr. Najjar handed me a blank sheet of paper that he had ripped out of his notebook and said, "Would you draw a clock for me and fill in all the numbers, 1 through 12?" I looked up at him with confusion. "As you remember it, Susannah. It does not have to be perfect."

I looked at the doctor and then back down at the paper. I held the pen loosely in my right hand, as if it were a foreign object. I first drew a circle, but it was lopsided and the lines were too squiggly. I asked for another sheet. He tore another out for me, and I tried again. This time a circle took shape. Because circle drawing is a type of procedural memory (one that was also still present in the famous amnesiac patient H.M.), that is, an over-learned practice, like tying shoes, patients have done it so many times before that they rarely get it wrong, so it didn't surprise him that I drew it with relative ease the second time. I outlined the circle once, twice, and then three times, an act called perseverative dysgraphia, a disorder in which a patient draws and redraws lines or letters. Dr. Najjar waited expectantly for the numbers.

"Now draw numbers on the clock."

I hesitated. He could see me straining to remember what a clock face looked like. I hunched over the paper and began to write. Methodically I wrote the numbers. Often I would get stuck on a number and draw it several times: more perseverative dysgraphia.

After a moment, Dr. Najjar looked down at the page and nearly applauded. I had squished all the numbers, 1 through 12, onto the right-hand side of the circle; it was a perfect specimen, with the twelve o'clock landing almost exactly where the six o'clock should have been.

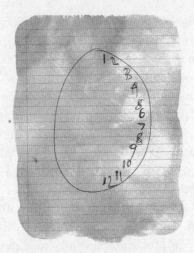

Re-creation of my clock drawing.

Dr. Najjar, beaming, grabbed the paper, showed it to my parents, and explained what this meant. They gasped with a combination of terror and hope. This was finally the clue that everyone was searching for. It didn't involve fancy machinery or invasive tests; it required only paper and pen. It had given Dr. Najjar concrete evidence that the right hemisphere of my brain was inflamed.

The healthy brain enables vision through a complex process involving both hemispheres. First, certain receptors are activated in the retina, and information passes through the eye and visual pathways until it reaches the primary visual cortex, located at the back of the brain, where it becomes one single perception, which the parietal and temporal lobes then process. The parietal lobes provide the person with the "where and when" of the image, situating us in time and space. The temporal lobe supplies the "who, what, and why," governing our ability to recognize names, feelings, and memories. But in a broken brain, where one hemisphere isn't working properly and the flow of information is obstructed, the visual world becomes lopsided.

Because the brain works contralaterally, meaning that the right hemisphere is responsible for the left field of vision and the left hemisphere is responsible for the right field of vision, my clock drawing, which had numbers drawn on only the right side, showed that the right hemisphere—responsible for seeing the left side of that clock—was compromised, to say the least. Visual neglect, however, is not blindness. The retinas are still active and still sending information to the visual cortex; it's just that the information is not being processed accurately in a way that enables us to "see" an image. A more accurate term for this, some doctors say, is visual indifference: the brain simply does not care about what's going on in the left side of its universe.

The clock test also helped explain another aspect of my illness that had largely been ignored: the numbness on the left side of my body that had since become a long-lost nonissue. The parietal lobe is also involved in sensation, and malfunction there could result in a feeling of numbness.

This single clock-drawing test answered so much: in addition to the numbness on the left side, it explained the paranoia, the seizures, and the hallucinations. It might even account for my imaginary bedbugs, since my "bites" occurred on my left arm. Ruling out schizoaffective disorder, postictal psychosis, and viral encephalitis and taking into account the high white blood cells in the lumbar puncture, Dr. Najjar had an epiphany: the inflammation was almost certainly the result of an autoimmune reaction, caused by my own body. But what type of autoimmune disease? There had been an autoimmune panel, which tests for only a small fraction of the hundred or so known autoimmune diseases, that had come back negative, so it couldn't be one of those. Dr. Najjar then recalled a series of cases in the recent medical literature about a rare autoimmune disease that affects mostly young women that had come out of the University of Pennsylvania. Could that be it?

There were other questions: How much inflammation? Was my brain salvageable? The only way to answer these questions was to do a brain biopsy, and he wasn't sure my parents would agree to one. No one liked the sound of a brain biopsy, which involved cutting out a small piece of my brain to study, but without quick intervention, my condition might not improve. The longer the problem continued without proper intervention, the worse my chances for returning to my former self became. As he mulled this over, he pulled at his mustache absentmindedly and paced around the room.

Finally, he sat down on the bed near me. He turned to my parents and said, "Her brain is on fire." He took my small hands into his large ones and leaned down to my eye level. "I'm going to do everything I can for you. I promise I will always be there for you."

For a moment, I seemed to come alive, he would later recall to me. I'll always regret that I remember nothing of this pivotal scene, one of the most important moments of my life.

Dr. Najjar saw tears gather at the corners of my eyes. I sat up and threw my arms around him. For him, it was another crucial moment in my case: he could sense that I was still in there, somewhere. But it was just a blip. After that outpouring, I lay back down and dozed off, exhausted by the brief display of emotion. But he knew I was there, and he would not give up on me. He motioned for my parents to follow him outside the room.

"Her brain is on fire," he repeated. They nodded, eyes wide. "Her brain is under attack by her own body."

CHAPTER 27

BRAIN BIOPSY

D r. Najjar's news didn't end there. "The next course of treatment, I feel, should be steroids, but we need to confirm the inflammation before moving on," he said.

"How?" my mother asked.

"There is a doctor at the University of Pennsylvania who specializes in autoimmune disease, and I believe he will have the answers we are looking for. Meanwhile," he paused, knowing my parents would not be pleased by what he was about to say, "there are several ways we can go with this. There are the steroids. There is plasmapheresis. There is IVIG."

My parents nodded again, in unison, entirely taken by this force of a man.

"But I think the best thing to do," he said, lowering his voice, "is to do a brain biopsy."

"What does that mean?" my mother asked quietly.

"We would need to look at her brain and take a small"—he put two fingers up and separated them by a centimeter—"piece of her brain."

My father bristled. "I don't know about that."

"I promise you that if it she were my child, I would do a brain biopsy. The risks of not doing it far outweigh the risks of doing it. The worst thing that can happen is that we end up in the same place we are now."

They didn't say a word.

"I want to do this Monday, Tuesday at the latest," he said. "But it is up to you. In the meantime, I will talk it over with the team and the surgeon. Let me think about it. And I will let you know."

As Dr. Najjar walked away, my mother whispered, "He's a real-life Dr. House."

Later that afternoon, Dr. Russo arrived to confirm to my parents that the team's decision was to move forward with a brain biopsy. My mom tried to remain calm, but she felt helpless. She motioned for Dr. Russo to join her outside the room in the hallway. She had so many questions for her, but all she could grasp on to were those two simple, bone-chilling words: brain biopsy. After weeks of maintaining a facade of composure, she had finally hit her breaking point and started to sob. Dr. Russo stood with her hands crossed over her chest and then reached out and ever so slightly touched my mother's arm.

"It's going to be fine," Dr. Russo said.

My mom wiped her tears and took a deep breath. "I better go back in."

When she returned, my dad threw her an accusatory glance. "We heard you," he said.

Despite his gruffness, as he would later write in his journal, he felt the same concerns as my mother: "The very sound of a brain biopsy scared me. I could hear my mother's voice telling me not to do it. I could hear her tell me to never let anyone mess with the brain. She had seen a lot of bad things happen as an RN and she didn't trust brain surgeons. I had to remind myself how long ago that was."

Depleted by the morning's events, the clock drawing, and the brain biopsy news, my dad walked across town from NYU to Thirty-Third Street, to catch the subway on Park Avenue South. Between First and Second Avenues, he spotted the Chapel of the Sacred Hearts of Jesus and Mary. Impulsively, he walked into the chapel, admiring the stained glass windows and the vibrant painting of an angel wrapping her arms around a broken man. He got on his knees and prayed.

That same afternoon, downtown in the Manhattan district attorney's office, my mom was doing something similar. She held hands with her secretary, Elsie, and her coworker Regina, who was also a Baptist minister. All three closed their eyes and held hands in a circle as Regina's voice rose high above them: "God, cure this young lady. God, hear us, hear our prayers. We pray for you to cure this girl and make her better. Hear our prayers. Please hear our prayers." My mom, a no-nonsense agnostic Jewish girl from the Bronx, now swears she felt the presence of God.

I was blissfully unaware of my parents' anguish. I texted my college friend Lindsey, who lived in St. Louis: "I'm getting a bri-annopsy!"

"What? What do you mean?" Lindsey wrote back, confused by the misspelling.

"They're taking a peece of my brain!"

My friend Zach, who was splitting cat-sitting duties with another coworker and friend, Ginger, called that day as well. I shared the news in the same manner that I would have told him what I had for lunch.

"I'm having a brain opsy," I said.

"Hold on, Susannah. They're doing surgery on your *brain*?" he asked, clearly concerned. It was the first time that someone had expressed to me directly how distressing the surgery sounded. I began to cry tears of fear and confusion and finally hung up, too upset to continue with the conversation.

———

It was Easter weekend. On Saturday, the surgeon's head nurse arrived to describe the preparation for the brain surgery. She seemed upbeat and managed to make the biopsy sound routine. This did not quell my father's fears. As she described where they were going to shave my head—the front part above my right fore-head about four inches in toward the crown—I listened impassively, and my dad was impressed by my dignity. It was only later that night that I began to break down. Seeing me upset made my dad cry too. Then he heard me laughing.

"You look funny when you cry," I giggled. Suddenly we were both laughing and crying. Through his tears, he reminded me of our motto.

"What's the slope of the line?"

"Um." I couldn't remember the answer.

"Positive. And what does that mean?"

"Um." I moved my arm upward, indicating progress.

"Right. Getting better every day."

The next day was Easter morning, and my dad brought me an Easter basket, the same basket he had given to me since I was a child, filled with chocolates and jellybeans. He was delighted to see me looking like a kid again, eyes wide, ready to pounce on the candy.

My parents arrived extra early on Monday morning, filled with both dread and excitement. For my part, I seemed unnaturally calm. Eventually an orderly, whom they thought looked like a Hells Angel, put me on a stretcher and wheeled me down into surgery. My parents hung back for a few seconds. Setting aside years of betrayal, emotional estrangement, and petty fights, they briefly exchanged a hug and a few quiet tears.

The OR was the embodiment of medicine on an industrial scale, a sterile place with doors snaking into dozens of operating theaters. Gone were the landscape paintings and soothing music; this was where the serious surgeries happened. We waited in the area immediately in front of the elevators, held back by large, clear vertical blinds. Everyone on the other side of the blinds wore surgical scrubs.

The neurosurgery resident came by to shave my head. The doctor shaved a good five-inch diameter section from my head, but, although I appeared fully conscious, I did not scream, call out, or cry. My dad again admired this strength, though it's possible I simply had no idea what was going on. I sat on the bed unfazed with my head wrapped in a towel, as if I had just received a spa treatment.

Fighting back tears, my dad knelt beside me.

"Remember what I told you. What is the strategy?"

"One step at a time."

"What is the slope of the line?"

"Positive."

Neurosurgeon Dr. Werner Doyle donned his surgical gown and prepped for surgery. He entered the operating room flanked by a scrub nurse, a circulating nurse, and an anesthesiologist. Despite the relative safety of this procedure, any number of things could still go wrong: they could have chosen the wrong location to dissect, and there is always a risk of infection or mistake with any type of surgery, especially the kinds involving the brain. But still, brain biopsies were simple compared to the more complex epilepsy surgeries that he had grown accustomed to performing over the years.

A new MRI had been loaded into his office computer and workstation, and it guided the surgeon through a process called frameless stereotactic neurosurgery, which involves the visual mapping of the brain in both three and two dimensions so that the surgeon can swiftly and accurately target one specific area of the brain—in this case, the right frontal cortex. He had already chosen an area, one without any large draining veins, farthest away from the parts of the brain responsible for motor functions. My gurney was rolled over to the operating table, my scalp shaved and cleaned. Then they put me under general anesthesia.

"Count down from 100," the anesthesiologist instructed.

"100 . . . 99 . . ."

As my eyes closed, they secured the head holder onto my temples to keep me still. With a scalpel, Dr. Doyle made an S-shape incision, 4 centimeters from the midline of the scalp over the right frontal region. The arm of the S extended just behind my hairline. He parted the skin with a sharp blade and gripped each side with retractors. Grasping a high-speed drill in his hands like a skillful carpenter, he pressed it down on the skull, making a "burr hole," or a 1-centimeter-diameter aperture through the bone of the skull. He then went over the burr hole with a craniotome, a bigger drill, grinding the bone into dust. He removed a 3-centimeter piece of the bone plate, exposing the dura, or the outermost, leathery, protective layer of the brain, and saved a section to send for testing along with the brain tissue.

With a fine #11 blade and a dissector, he cut several cubes of tissue, equaling about 1 cubic centimeter in volume, which included white matter (strands of nerve fibers) and gray matter (the cell bodies of neurons). He set aside specimens for future studies and an extra sample to be frozen in case other tests were needed. He swabbed the brain matter and stopped the blood flow using cottonoids, highly absorbent synthetic fibers.

He then very carefully stitched a dura graft onto the outer layer of the brain, suturing it together, and then reattached the bone plate. He pushed the plate to one side, butting it up against the existing bone so that it would fuse, and then secured the plate using screws and a small metal plate. He ended the procedure by returning the outer layer of skin to its original position, and closing the scalp with metal staples. The whole procedure took four hours.

"Count down from 100," a disembodied voice says.
"100 . . . 99 . . . 98 . . ."
Darkness.
Blink. Blink. Blink. "I'm still awake."
Darkness.
A crowded recovery room. I'm alone. There's a family to the right of me, surrounding another patient. Where are my parents?
Then I see them. Mom and Dad. I can't move.
Then Stephen and Allen. I try to raise my arm slightly to wave; it feels as heavy as a fifty-pound weight.

Darkness.

"Thirsty." My voice is hoarse. "Thirsty."

"Here," a brusque nurse says, shoving a water-soaked sponge into my mouth. The texture is unpleasant but the water is a godsend. I suck and suck. "Thirsty." She shoves another one in my mouth. I hear the parents beside me feeding their kid ice chips. I raise my arm. I want some. A male nurse approaches. "Ice." He brings me a few ice chips and places them on my tongue. I can hear the female nurse telling him not to give me water. "She can't have any water. Just ignore her."

"Water, water," I moan.

She approaches. "I'm sorry but you can't have any more."

"I'm going to tell everyone how you treated me. I'm going to tell everyone when I get out of here."

"What did you say?" Her tone scares me.

"Nothing."

Darkness.

I'm in a claustrophobic one-person room. I have to pee. I have to pee. I push. My catheter comes undone and the urine sprays all over the bed. I call out. A nurse comes in.

"I peed."

Another nurse joins her. They turn me on my left side, remove the bedding, wash me with warm towels, and spritz me with something. Then they turn me over to the right side and repeat. It feels nice. But I can't move. I push hard with my brain, trying to wiggle my toes. I push so hard that I get a headache. My toes don't move.

"I can't move my legs," I call out.

Many hours after the surgery, around 11:00 p.m., a nurse informed my dad, who had chosen to wait for news while everyone else went home at the staff's insistence, that I had been moved from the recovery room into the ICU. They didn't invite him in to see me, but he wandered into the unit anyway, unaccompanied. The floor consisted of a handful of bays, one patient in each. There were nurses everywhere, but no one even looked twice at him. He peeked into each bay until he spotted me.

There I was, semiconscious, propped up on pillows with my head wrapped in white gauze like some kind of sick Persian princess. I was attached to monitors and machines that beeped and groaned and had been wrapped up in nude compression stockings to keep my blood pressure normal. When he caught my eye, I instantly recognized him, which didn't always happen. We hugged.

"The worst is behind you, Susannah."

"Where's Mom?" I asked.

"She will see you tomorrow," he said. He could tell I was upset that my mother hadn't come, even though it had been the right decision for her to go home that night. Then: "I can't feel my legs, Dad." I sounded convinced.

"Are you sure, Susannah?" my dad asked, turning white with fear. This had been the worry all along, that they would do permanent damage by messing with my brain.

"Yes. I can't move them."

My dad immediately called in a young resident, who came in and examined me, then rushed me out for an emergency MRI. My dad silently hurried beside the gurney, holding my hand until the MRI technician whisked me into the room, telling my dad to wait. In those thirty minutes, he would later sigh, he lost five years off his life. But the young resident eventually emerged to tell him that everything looked fine.

My dad stayed with me until I fell asleep. Then he went home and slid into bed, prayed, and fell into a restless slumber.

CHAPTER 28

SHADOWBOXER

After the surgery, I was reassigned to a shared room on the epilepsy unit. My roommate, a woman in her early thirties, suffered from seizures induced during alcohol consumption (though seizures occur commonly with alcohol withdrawal, sometimes drinking can induce seizures). She was constantly begging the staff to allow her to drink some wine so that they could record the seizure. They refused.

The results of the brain biopsy confirmed what the team had expected: my brain was inflamed. Dr. Najjar's slides showed armies of angry inflammatory cells from my immune system attacking nerve cells in the brain, a signature of encephalitis.

There was a time, not so long ago, when neurologists believed that the brain was immunoprivileged, meaning it was completely separate from the immune system's lymphocytes; now doctors use the careful phrasing "immuno-different." The blood-brain barrier (BBB) is a dense patchwork quilt of vessels that serve as gates, regulating the passage of substances, like bacteria, chemicals, and drugs, from the blood to the brain. Researchers have discovered that the BBB does allow for certain B-cells and T-cells to squeeze through, in a process called diapedesis, to do regular "checkups." But this was no routine checkup. The immune cells it had let through, which were supposed to protect the body, were in mid-blitz. This was the evidence Dr. Najjar had needed: I was in the grip of some kind of autoimmune disease.

Now that they had a hazy diagnosis, the doctors could move ahead with the first phase of treatment, intravenous steroids, a form of immunotherapy that suppresses inflammation created by the body's immune system. A clear plastic bag of Solu-Medrol, an IV steroid, hung beside my bed for three days of intensive therapy. It was administered every six hours on an IV pump. These steroids, called corticosteroids, subdue the inflammation and quiet the immune system, which in turn quells future inflammation. As the steroids seeped into my system, they switched off inflammatory chemicals called cytokines. Dr. Najjar approved the highest dosage possible for three days. Then he would convert me to 60 milligrams of the oral steroid prednisone, which would continue, more gently, to quell the inflammation over time.

Because corticosteroids interact with blood-sugar levels, among other things, I developed a temporary form of type II diabetes. Though the doctors changed my menu, providing only sugar-free Jell-O as a sweet snack, my parents remained oblivious to the dangers of my Easter jellybeans, as I continued to munch away. Since I was placed on bed rest following surgery, the nurses applied thigh-high compression boots, which blow up and deflate, pumping blood through my legs and mimicking the act of contracting and expanding during physical activity. But they made my legs itchy and sweaty, as I explained to anyone who would listen, and I kicked them off every night.

Despite the new intensive steroid treatment, my condition did not seem to improve right away. In fact, it worsened; the abnormal nightly movements and undefined panic attacks increased. My father wrote about my continued difficulties in the logbook that he and my mom shared: "She had a strange smirking expression on her face. She tensed up," he wrote. "Arms stretched out straight, grimace, tenseness, shakes."

But I could still pull myself together for visitors. Hannah arrived soon after the surgery and stifled a laugh when she saw my strange white turban of bandages.

I was a good sport about it. "I'm going to be bald!" I said, smiling, and popped an Easter jellybean into my mouth.

"What do you mean? Did they shave your scalp?"

"Bald!"

"Maybe you need Propecia." We both cracked up.

EEG video, April 12, 8:12 a.m., 7 minutes

I'm wearing a white surgical cap, reclining with my legs folded over as if I'm sunbathing. My pink backpack containing the EEG box rests on my lower stomach. I get up and walk to the door. My movements are halting and painfully slow. My left arm is outstretched.

"Would that be the little green button?" my mother asks a nurse from off-camera, referring to the seizure/event button tied to the bedside rail. She enters the frame and sits by the window.

I get back into bed. My mother gets up and hovers over me and then pushes the nurse's button. Nurse Edward arrives moments later and starts a neurological exam, miming the action he wants me to follow, extending his arms out. Gradually I follow his lead. He taps on my left index finger and tells me to close my eyes and touch it to my face. After a moment, I do. He repeats it on the other side.

When Edward leaves, I reach for the sheets. It takes a full ten seconds for me to lie down. Meanwhile, my mother looks nervous. She checks her purse, crosses and uncrosses her legs, all the while keeping an eye on me.

End of video.

By our third night in the shared room, the woman next to me had a seizure. Somehow she had convinced the medical staff to allow her to drink wine. Since they had what they needed, a physical recording of a seizure, she was released shortly thereafter.

CHAPTER 29
DALMAU'S DISEASE

Dr. Russo arrived later that day to explain which diseases they could now tick off the list of possibilities, including hyperthyroidism, lymphoma, and Devic's disease, a rare disease similar symptomatically to multiple sclerosis. They still suspected that I had been exposed to hepatitis, which can cause encephalitis, but they didn't have proof.

After the conversation, my mother followed Dr. Russo into the hallway. "So what do *you* think it is?" my mom prodded.

"Actually, Dr. Najjar and I have a bet going."

"What kind of a bet?"

"Well, Dr. Najjar thinks the inflammation is caused by autoimmune encephalitis; I think it's paraneoplastic syndrome." When my mother pressed for more details, Dr. Russo explained that paraneoplastic syndrome is a consequence of an underlying cancer, most often associated with lung, breast, or ovarian cancer. The symptoms—psychosis, catatonia, and so forth—are not associated with the cancer but with the immune system's response to it. As the body gears up to attack the tumor, it sometimes begins to target healthy parts of the body, such as the spine or the brain. "I think because of her history of melanoma, it makes sense," Dr. Russo concluded.

This was not what my mother wanted to hear. Cancer had always been the greatest fear, the word she dared not utter. Now this doctor was tossing it off casually as part of a bet.

—————

Meanwhile, two plastic tubes, placed securely in Styrofoam boxes, had arrived at the University of Pennsylvania, transported in a refrigerator in the back of a FedEx truck; one contained transparent cerebrospinal fluid, as clear as unfiltered water, and another held blood, which started to look like dehydrated urine as, over time, the red blood cells dropped to the bottom. The test tubes were coded 0933, labeled with my initials, SC, and placed in a negative-80 degree freezer waiting for the lab to conduct its tests. They were addressed to the lab run by neuro-oncologist Dr. Josep Dalmau, whom Dr. Najjar had mentioned during his first visit and whom Dr. Russo had since e-mailed to ask if he would take a look at my case.

Four years earlier, in 2005, Dr. Dalmau had been the senior author on a paper in the neuroscience journal *Annals of Neurology* that focused on four young women who had developed prominent psychiatric symptoms and encephalitis. All had white blood cells in their cerebrospinal fluid, confusion, memory problems, hallucinations, delusions, and difficulty breathing, and they all had tumors called teratomas in their ovaries. But the most remarkable finding was that all four patients had similar antibodies that appeared to be reacting against specific areas of the brain, mainly the hippocampus. Something about the combination of the tumor and the antibodies was making these women very sick.

Dr. Dalmau had noticed a pattern in these four women; now he had to learn more about the antibody itself. He and his research team began to work night and day on an elaborate immunohistrochemistry experiment involving frozen sections of rat brains, which had been sliced into paper-thin pieces and then exposed to the cerebrospinal fluid of those four sick women. The hope was that the antibodies from the cerebrospinal fluid would bind directly to some receptors in the rat brain and reveal a characteristic design. It took eight months of tinkering before a pattern finally emerged.

Dr. Dalmau had prepared the rat brain slides all the same, placing a small amount of cerebrospinal fluid from each of the four patients on each. Twenty-four hours later:

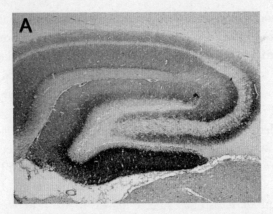

A: Section of rat brain in the hippocampus that shows the reactivity of the cerebrospinal fluid of a patient with anti-NMDAR encephalitis. The brown staining corresponds to the patient's antibodies that have bound to the NMDA receptors.

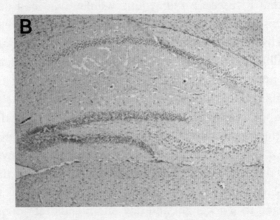

B: A similar section of hippocampus of an individual without NMDA receptor antibodies.

Four beautiful images, like cave drawings or abstract seashell patterns, revealed the antibodies' binding to the naked eye. "It was a moment of great excitement," Dr. Dalmau later recalled. "Everything had been negative. Now we became totally positive that all four not only had the same illness, but the same antibody."

He had clarified that the pattern of reactivity was more intense in the hippocampus of the rat brain, but this was only the beginning. A far more difficult question now arose: Which receptors were these antibodies targeting? Through a combination of trial and error, plus a few educated guesses about which receptors are most common in the hippocampus, Dr. Dalmau and his colleagues eventually identified the target. Using a kidney cell line bought from a commercial lab that came with no receptors on their surfaces at all, a kind of "blank slate," his lab introduced DNA sequences that direct the cells to make certain types of receptors, allowing the lab to control which receptors were available for binding. Dalmau chose to have them express only NMDA receptors, after figuring out that those were the most likely to have been present in high volume in the hippocampus. Sure enough, the antibodies in the cerebrospinal fluid of the four patients bound to the cells. There was his answer: the culprits were NMDA-receptor-seeking antibodies.

NMDA (N-methyl-D-aspartate acid) receptors are vital to learning, memory, and behavior, and they are a main staple of our brain chemistry. If these are incapacitated, mind and body fail. NMDA receptors are located all over the brain, but the majority are concentrated on neurons in the hippocampus, the brain's primary learning and memory center, and in the frontal lobes, the seat of higher functions and personality. These receptors receive instructions from chemicals called neurotransmitters. All neurotransmitters carry only one of two messages: they can either "excite" a cell, encouraging it to fire an electrical impulse, or "inhibit" a cell, which hinders it from firing. These simple conversations between neurons are at the root of everything we do, from sipping a glass of wine to writing a newspaper lead.

In those unfortunate patients with Dr. Dalmau's anti-NMDA-receptor encephalitis, the antibodies, normally a force for good in the body, had become treasonous persona non grata in the brain. These receptor-seeking antibodies planted their death kiss on the surface of a neuron, handicapping the neuron's receptors, making them unable to send and receive those important chemical signals. Though researchers are far from fully understanding how NMDA receptors (and their corresponding neurons) affect and alter behavior, it's clear that when they are compromised the outcome can be disastrous, even deadly.

Still, a few experiments have offered up some clues as to their importance. Decrease NMDA receptors by, say, 40 percent, and you might get psychosis; decrease them by 70 percent, and you have catatonia. In "knockout mice" without NMDA receptors at all, even the most basic life functions are impossible: most die within ten hours of birth due to respiratory failure. Mice with a very small number of NMDA receptors don't learn to suckle, and they simply starve to death within a day or so. Those mice with at least 5 percent of their NMDA receptors intact survive, but exhibit abnormal behavior and strange social and sexual interactions. Mice with half their receptors in working order also live, but they show memory deficits and abnormal social relationships.

As a result of this additional research, in 2007, Dr. Dalmau and his colleagues presented another paper, now introducing his new class of NMDA-receptor-seeking diseases to the world. This second article identified twelve women with the same profile of neurological symptoms, which could now be called a syndrome. They all had teratomas, and almost all of them were young women. Within a year after publication, one hundred more patients had been diagnosed; not all of them had ovarian teratomas and not all of them were young women (some were men and many were children), enabling Dr. Dalmau to do an even more thorough study on the newly discovered, but nameless, disease.

"Why not name it the Dalmau disease?" people often asked him. But he didn't think "Dalmau disease" sounded right, and it was no longer customary to name a disease after its discoverer. "I didn't think that would be wise. It's not very humble." He shrugged.

By the time I was a patient at NYU, Dr. Dalmau had fine-tuned his approach, designing two tests that could swiftly and accurately diagnose the disease. As soon as he received my samples, he could test the spinal fluid. If he found that I had anti-NMDA-receptor autoimmune encephalitis, it would make me the 217th person worldwide to be diagnosed since 2007. It just begged the question: If it took so long for one of the best hospitals in the world to get to this step, how many other people were going untreated, diagnosed with a mental illness or condemned to a life in a nursing home or a psychiatric ward?

CHAPTER 30
RHUBARB

B y my twenty-fifth day in the hospital, two days after the biopsy, with a preliminary diagnosis in sight, my doctors thought it was a good time to officially assess my cognitive skills to record a baseline. This test would be a fulcrum, a turning point, that would measure what kind of progress they could expect in the future through the various stages of treatment. Beginning on the afternoon of April 15, a speech pathologist and a neuropsychologist visited me for two days in a row, each for separate assessments.

The speech pathologist, Karen Gendal, did the first assessment, starting with basic questions: "What's your name?" "How old are you?" "Are you a woman?" "Do you live in California?" "Do you live in New York?" "Do you peel a banana before eating it?" and so forth. I was able to answer all of these questions, though I did so slowly. But when she asked the more open-ended question "Why are you in the hospital?" I could not explain. (To be fair, the doctors didn't know either, but I could not provide even the basics.)

After some spotty and tangential answers, I finally said, "I can't get my ideas from my head out." She nodded: this was a typical response for people suffering from aphasia, a language impairment related to brain injury. I also had something called dysarthria, a motor speech impairment caused by a weakness in the muscles of the face, throat, or vocal cords.

Gendal asked me to stick out my tongue, which trembled from the effort. It had a reduced range of motion on both sides, which was contributing to my inability to articulate.

"Would you smile for me?"

I tried, but my facial muscles were so weak that no smile came. She wrote down "hypo-aroused," a medical term for lethargic, and also noted that I was not fully alert. When I did talk, the words came out without any emotional register.

She moved on to cognitive abilities. Holding up her pen, she asked, "What is this?"

"Ken," I answered. This, again, wasn't too unusual for someone at my level of impairment. They call it *phonemic paraphasia,* where you substitute one word for another that sounds similar.

When she asked me to write my name, I painstakingly drew out an "S," tracing the letter multiple times before moving on to the "U," where I did the same. It took several minutes for me to write my name. "Okay, would you write this sentence out for me: 'Today is a nice day.'"

I drew out the letters, retracing each of them several times and misspelling some words. My handwriting was so poor that Gendal could hardly make out the sentence.

She wrote her impression in the chart: "It is difficult to determine at just two days post-operation to what extent communication deficits are language-based versus medication or cognitive. Clearly communication function is dramatically reduced from pre-morbid level when this patient was working as a successful journalist for a local paper." In other words, there seemed to be a dramatic change between the person I had been and the person I was now, but it was difficult at the time to distinguish my problems understanding from my inability to communicate—and whether these would persist in the long or short term.

Later the next morning, neuropsychologist Chris Morrison arrived with her auburn hair piled high on her head and green-flecked hazel eyes flashing. She was there to test me on something called the Wechsler Abbreviated Scale of Intelligence, as well as other tests, that are used to diagnose a number of things, from attention deficit disorder to traumatic brain injuries. But when she entered the room, I was so unresponsive she wasn't even sure that I could see her.

"What is your name?" Dr. Morrison began brightly, walking me through the basic orienting questions that by now I had been conditioned to answer correctly. Her next stage of questions assessed attention, processing speed, and working memory, which she compared to a computer's random access memory (RAM), as in, "How many programs you can have open all at once—how many things you can keep in your head at once and spit back out."

Dr. Morrison provided me with a random assortment of single-digit numbers, 1 through 9, and asked me to repeat them to her. Once we got up to five digits, I had to stop, though seven is the normal limit for people of my age and intelligence.

Next, she tested the word-retrieval process, to see how well I was able to access my "memory bank." "I'd like you to name as many fruits and vegetables as possible," she said, starting a sixty-second timer.

"Apples," I began. Apples are a common fruit to start with, and of course they had been on my mind a lot lately.

"Carrots."

"Pears."

"Bananas."

Pause.

"Rhubarb."

Dr. Morrison chuckled inwardly at this one. The minute was over. I had come up with five fruits and vegetables; a healthy individual could name over twenty. Dr. Morrison believed that I knew plenty more examples; the problem seemed to be retrieving them.

She then showed me a series of cards with everyday objects on them. I could name only five of the ten, missing examples like kite and pliers, though I struggled as if the words were on the tip of my tongue.

Dr. Morrison then tested my ability to view and process the external world. There are many different things that must come together for a person to accurately perceive an object. To see a desk, for example, first we see lines that come together at angles, then color, then contrast, then depth; all of that information goes into the memory bank, which labels it with a word and, depending on the object, an emotion (to a journalist, a desk might elicit guilty feelings about missed deadlines, for example). To track this set of skills, she had me compare the size and shape of various angles. I scored on the low end of average on these, well enough for Dr. Morrison to move on to more difficult tasks. She introduced a set of red and white blocks and placed them on the foldout tray in front of me. She then showed me a picture of how the blocks should be arranged and asked me to re-create the picture with a timer running.

I stared at the pictures and then back at the blocks, moved them into a pattern that had nothing to do with the picture, and looked back at the picture for reference. I fiddled with the blocks some more, getting nowhere, but refused to give up. Morrison wrote down "tenacious in her attempts." I seemed to realize I wasn't getting it right, which frustrated me deeply. It was clear that, for all my other impairments, I knew that I was not functioning at the level I was used to.

The next step was for me to copy down complex geometric designs on graph paper, but my abilities here were so weak that Dr. Morrison decided to stop altogether. I was flustered, and she worried that moving forward would only make me feel worse. Dr. Morrison was convinced that I was very much aware, despite the cognitive issues, of what I could no longer do. In her review later that day, she marked cognitive therapy as "highly recommended."

CHAPTER 31
THE BIG REVEAL

Later that afternoon, my dad had been trying to interest me in a game of gin rummy when Dr. Russo and the team arrived.

"Mr. Cahalan," she said. "We have some positive test results."

He dropped the playing cards on the floor and grabbed his notebook. Dr. Russo explained that they'd heard back from Dr. Dalmau with a confirmation of the diagnosis. Her words flew at him like shrapnel—bang, bang, bang: *NMDA, antibody, tumor, chemotherapy.* He fought to pay close attention, but there was one key part of the explanation that he could hold on to: my immune system had gone haywire and had begun attacking my brain.

"I'm sorry," he interrupted the barrage. "What is the name again?"

He wrote the letters "NMDA" in his block lettering:

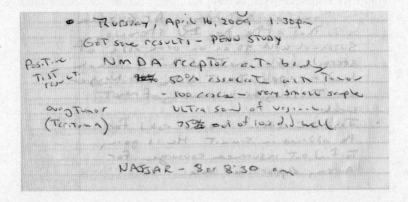

Anti-NMDA-receptor encephalitis, Dr. Russo explained, is a multistage disease that varies wildly in its presentation as it progresses. For 70 percent of patients, the disorder begins innocuously, with normal flulike symptoms: headaches, fever, nausea, and vomiting, though it's unclear if patients initially contract a virus related to the disease or if these symptoms are a result of the disease itself. Typically, about two weeks after the initial flulike symptoms, psychiatric issues, which include anxiety, insomnia, fear, grandiose delusions, hyperreligiosity, mania, and paranoia, take hold. Because the symptoms are psychiatric, most patients seek out mental health professionals first. Seizures crop up in 75 percent of patients, which is fortunate if only because they get the patient out of the psychologist's chair and into a neurologist's office. From there, language and memory deficits arise, but they are often overshadowed by the more dramatic psychiatric symptoms.

My father sighed with relief. He felt comforted by a name, any name, to explain what had happened to me, even if he didn't quite understand what it all meant. Everything she said was matching up perfectly to my case, including abnormal facial tics, lip smacking, and tongue jabbing, along with synchronized and rigid body movements. Patients also often develop autonomic symptoms, she continued: blood pressure and heart rate that vacillate between too high and too low—again, just like my case. She hardly needed to point out that I had now entered the catatonic stage, which marks the height of the disease but also precedes breathing failure, coma, and sometimes death. The doctors seemed to have caught it just in time.

When Dr. Russo began to explain that there are treatments that have been proven to reverse the course of the disease, my father nearly sank to his knees and thanked God right there in the hospital room. Still, Dr. Russo cautioned, even once you have a diagnosis, there are still substantial question marks. Though 75 percent of patients recover fully or maintain only mild side effects, over 20 percent remain permanently disabled and 4 percent die anyway, even despite a swift diagnosis. And those aforementioned "mild" side effects might mean the difference between the old me and a new Susannah, one who might not have the humor, vitality, or drive that I did before. *Mild* is a vague and undefined term.

"About 50 percent of the time, the disease is instigated by an ovarian tumor, called a teratoma, but in the other 50 percent of cases, the cause is never discovered," Dr. Russo continued.

My dad looked at her quizzically. *What the hell is a teratoma?*

It was probably best that he didn't know. When this type of tumor was identified in the late 1800s, a German doctor christened it "teratoma" from the Greek *teraton,* which means monster. These twisted cysts were a source of fascination even when there was no name for them: the first description dates back to a Babylonian text from 600 B.C. These masses of tissue range in size from microscopic to fist sized (or even bigger) and contain hair, teeth, bone, and sometimes even eyes, limbs, and brain tissue. They are often located in the reproductive organs, brain, skull, tongue, and neck and resemble pus-soaked hairballs. They are like those hairy, toothy creatures in the 1980s horror film franchise *Critters.* The only good news is that they are usually—but not always—benign.

"We will need to do a transvaginal exam to see if there are any signs of tumors," said Dr. Russo. "We'll also check her over to see if there's any link with her history of melanoma. If so, we'll have to move on with chemotherapy."

"Chemotherapy." My father repeated the word in the hope that she had gotten it wrong. But she hadn't.

My dad looked over at me. I had been staring off to the side, disassociated from the exchange, not seeming to gauge the magnitude of the moment. Suddenly, though, at the word *chemotherapy,* my chest began heaving, and I let out a deep sigh. Tears streamed down my face. My dad ran from his chair and threw his arms around me. I continued to sob without saying a word, as Dr. Russo waited quietly while he rocked me. He couldn't tell if I understood what was going on or if I was just attuned to the amplified electricity in the room.

"This is killing me," I said, my voice high yet unemotional, despite the sobs. "I'm dying in here."

"I know, I know," he said. With my head in his arms, he could smell the glue on my hair. "We're going to get you out of here."

After a few moments, my sobs stopped, and I lay back on the bed, my head against the pillow, staring straight ahead. Quietly, Dr. Russo continued. "Overall, this is good news, Mr. Cahalan. Dr. Najjar believes that there is a possibility that Susannah could get back as much as 90 percent of her former self."

"We could get her back?"

"There seems to be a strong possibility."

"I want to go home," I said.

"We're working on doing just that," Dr. Russo replied with a smile.

—∽∽—

Over the weeks, I had gone from being a notoriously difficult patient to a favorite, the ward's "interesting consult" for a host of attending doctors, interns, and residents hoping to catch a glimpse of the girl with the unknown disease. Now that we had a diagnosis that had never before been seen at NYU, young MDs, hardly a day older than me, stared at me as if I were a caged animal in a zoo and made muffled assessments, pointing at me and craning their heads as more experienced doctors gave a rundown of the syndrome. The next morning, as my father fed me oatmeal and chopped-up bananas, a group of residents and medical students arrived. The young man leading the group of nascent MDs introduced my case as if I weren't in the room.

"This is a very interesting one," he said, leading a gang of about six others into the room. "She has what is called anti-NMDA-receptor autoimmune encephalitis."

The group ogled me and a few even let out a few quiet "ooohs" and "ahhhs." My father gritted his teeth and tried to ignore them.

"In about 50 percent of the cases, there is a teratoma in the ovaries. If this is the case, this patient may have her ovaries removed as a precaution."

As the spectators nodded their heads, I caught this somehow, and began to cry.

My father bolted from his seat. This was the first time he had heard anything about my ovaries being removed, and he certainly didn't want either of us hearing it from this kid. A born fighter and a strong man for his age (or for any other age), my dad bum-rushed the scrawny young physician and pointed a finger in his face.

"You get the fuck out of here right now!" His voice bounced around the hospital room. "Never come back. Get the fuck out of the room."

The young doctor's confidence deflated. Instead of apologizing, he waved his hand, urging the other interns to follow him toward the door, and made his escape.

"Forget you heard that, Susannah," my dad said. "They have no idea what the hell they're talking about."

CHAPTER 32

90 PERCENT

That same day, a dermatologist arrived and conducted a full-body skin exam to check for melanoma, which took about thirty minutes because my body is covered in moles. But after a thorough search, the dermatologist concluded that, happily, there was no sign of melanoma. That evening, they wheeled me down, yet again, to the second-floor radiology department, where they would conduct an ultrasound of my pelvis in search of a teratoma.

I am awakened, even though I hadn't been asleep. I had imagined this moment: the time when I would find out the gender of my child. Momentarily, I think, "I hope it's a boy." But the feeling passes. I would be happy with either a girl or a boy. I can feel the cool metal of the transducer against my belly. My chest wall leaps up into my throat in reaction to the cold. It was almost exactly how I imagined it to be. But then again not at all.

Distraught by the first ultrasound, I refused a transvaginal one, the more invasive pelvic examination. Still, even from the imperfect first test, there was good news: no sign of a teratoma. The bad news was that, ironically, teratomas were *good* news, because those with them tend to improve faster than people without them, for reasons researchers still don't understand.

Dr. Najjar arrived the next morning alone and greeted my parents as if they were old friends. Now that they had identified the disease, and knew that there was no teratoma, it was time to figure out what treatment could save me. If he miscalculated, I might never recover. He had spent the night deliberating about what to do, waking up in sweats and rambling to his wife. He had finally decided to act with abandon. He didn't want to wait for things to worsen; I was already too close to the edge. He delivered the plan of action while tugging at the corners of his mustache, deep in thought.

"We're going to put her on an aggressive treatment of steroids, IVIG treatment, and plasmapheresis," he said. Although he had a terrific bedside manner, sometimes he expected his patients to follow him as if they were trained neurologists.

"What will these all do?" my mother asked.

"It's a three-pronged attack, no stoned turned," Dr. Najjar said, missing the English idiom. "We're going to reduce the body's inflammation with steroids. Then flush the body of the antibodies with plasmapheresis, and further reduce and neutralize the antibodies with IVIG. It leaves no room for error."

"When will she be able to go home?" my dad asked.

"As far as I'm concerned, she could leave tomorrow," Dr. Najjar replied. "The steroids could be taken orally. She could return to the hospital for plasma exchange, and the IVIG treatment, if the insurance company approved it, could be done with a nurse at home. With all these treatments I believe that it's likely Susannah will get back to 90 percent."

Though I don't remember the diagnosis, my parents tell me that when I heard this my demeanor changed, and I seemed bolstered by the news that I would be returning home soon. Dr. Russo noted in my chart that I appeared "brighter," my speech "improved."

Home. I was going home.

The next morning, Saturday, April 18, I was finally discharged. I had been in the hospital for twenty-eight days. Many of the nurses—some of whom had washed me, others who had injected me with sedatives, and a few of whom had fed me when I could not feed myself—came to say their good-byes. Nurses seldom find out how a patient fares after she leaves the hospital, and I was still in a particularly bad place. A small, hunched-over man entered the room holding papers. He had secured an at-home nurse to tend to me and had recommended a clinic where I could receive full-time rehab. My mother took the papers, but only absentmindedly flipped through them; she would address these later. For now, we were going home, and that was all that mattered.

My mom, my dad, Allen, Stephen, and my college friend Lindsey, who had flown in from St. Louis the day before, all grabbed my possessions—stuffed animals, DVDs, clothes, books, and toiletries—and crammed them in clear plastic NYU "Patient's Belongings" bags; they left behind the flowers and magazines. A transport staff worker helped me into a wheelchair as my mom placed slip-on flats on my feet. It was the first time I had worn shoes in a month.

The night before, my dad had made a sign thanking the nurses for their support. He posted it near the elevators:

THANK YOU

On behalf of our daughter Susannah Cahalan, we would like very much to thank the entire staff of the epilepsy floor at NYU Medical Center. We came to you with a difficult and desperate situation, and you responded with skill and compassion. Susannah is a wonderful young woman who deserved your hard work. Her mother and I will forever be in your debt. I cannot think of more meaningful work than what you do every day.

Rhona Nack
Tom Cahalan

My prognosis was still unclear—the projection was only "fair"—and no one could say with any certainty if I would ever get to that optimistic "90 percent," or if I would ever regain any semblance of my former self. But they had a plan. First, I would continue to see Dr. Najjar every other Wednesday. Second, I would get a full-body positron emission tomography scan (PET scan) that creates a three-dimensional image of the body, which is different from MRIs and CT scans because it shows the body in the process of functioning. Third, I would be enrolled in cognitive and speech rehabilitation, and they would arrange for a twenty-four-hour nurse to care for me. Fourth, I would take oral steroids, receive plasma-exchange treatment, and get several more infusions of IVIG. But the doctors were aware that even months after the disease has run its course and immunosuppressants have been worked into the system, antibodies can still persist, making recovery a painful march of two steps forward, one step back.

They gave my mother a list of the medications I would now be taking: prednisone; Ativan, an antianxiety drug used to treat and prevent signs of catatonia; Geodon for psychosis; Trileptal for seizures; Labetalol for high blood pressure; Nexium to deal with the acid reflux caused by the steroids; and Colace for the constipation caused by the combination of all the drugs. Still, in the back of everyone's mind was that 4 percent mortality figure. Even with all of this, with all the proper intervention, people still died. Sure, they had a name for my illness and actions we could all take, but there was still a long uncertain journey ahead.

Stephen, Lindsey, and I filed into Allen's Subaru. When I had been admitted in early March, it was still winter; now it was springtime in New York. We drove back to Summit in silence. Allen turned on the radio, tuning it to a local lite FM station. Lindsey looked over at me to see if I recognized the song.

"Don't go breaking my heart," a man's voice started.

"I couldn't if I tried," a woman's voice returned.

This had been my go-to karaoke song in college in St. Louis. At this point, Lindsey doubted I would remember it.

I began bopping my head out of rhythm, my arms at rigid right angles. I swung my elbows front to back like I was awkwardly cross-country skiing. Was this one of my weird seizure-like moments, or was I dancing to an old favorite? Lindsey couldn't tell.

CHAPTER 33

HOMECOMING

My mom's house in Summit looked particularly striking that spring day, my homecoming. The front lawn was lush with fresh green grass, white azaleas, and the blooms of pinkish-purple rhododendrons and yellow daffodils. The sun beamed down on the aged oak trees that shaded the maroon door at the entrance-way to the stone-front colonial. It was gorgeous, but no one could tell if I even noticed. I certainly don't remember it. I just stared ahead, making that constant chewing motion with my mouth as Allen swerved into the driveway of the place I had called home most of my young adult life.

The first thing that I wanted to do was take a real shower. There were still clumps of glue in my scalp that looked like pebble-sized pieces of dandruff, and I still had the metal staples from the surgery, so I could not be too vigorous with my washing. My mother offered to help, but I refused, determined to do this small thing on my own, at last.

After a half hour, Lindsey headed upstairs to check on me. Through the opening in my bedroom door, she could see me sitting on the bed, freshly showered, with my legs flexed rigidly off the side, fidgeting with the zipper on my black hoodie. I was struggling to connect the zipper with the pull. Lindsey watched for a moment, unsure of what to do; she didn't want to embarrass me by knocking on the door and offering aid, because she knew I didn't like to be babied. But when she saw me go limp, drop the zipper, and begin to sob out of frustration, she headed into the room. She sat down beside me and said, "Here, let me help," zipping up my hoodie in one fluid motion.

. . .

Later that evening, Stephen cooked a pasta dinner as a quiet celebration for my return. Allen and my mom left the house so that
the three of us could have some alone time. My mother was so
relieved that they finally had a name for what ailed me that she
had truly convinced herself the worst was behind us.

After dinner, we sat outside on the back patio. Lindsey and
Stephen made small talk while I stared ahead, as if I didn't hear
them. But when they lit cigarettes, I got up without a word and
walked inside.

"Is she okay?" Lindsey asked.

"Yes, I think she's just adjusting. We should give her a moment
alone."

*They are smoking together. Who knows what else they'll do
together.*

*I grab the home phone. For some reason, I can't remember
my mother's number, so I look it up in my cell phone. Ring, ring,
ring, ring.*

*"You've reached Rhona Nack. Please leave a message after the
beep." BEEP.*

*"Mom," I whisper. "He's going to leave me for her. Please
come home. Please come home and stop them."*

*I pace around and watch him from the kitchen window that
looks out on the patio. He catches my eye and waves. Why does
he want to be with a sick girl? What is he doing here with me? I
look at him waving, certain that I have lost him forever.*

When my mom listened to the voice mail, she panicked: I was
becoming psychotic again. Because Dr. Najjar was often difficult
to reach, she dialed Dr. Arslan's private number, which he had
given her the day before we left the hospital. She was worried that
NYU had let me go home too soon.

"She's acting paranoid," she said. "She believes that her boy-friend is going to run off with her best friend."

This concerned Dr. Arslan. "I'm worried that she may be reen-tering a psychotic state. I would give her an extra dose of Ativan to calm her for the night and then check in with me tomorrow." In my case, though, the return to psychotic behavior was actually a sign of improvement, because the stages of recovery often occur in reverse order: I had passed through psychosis before I got to cata-tonia, and now I had to pass through it again on my road back to normality. Dr. Arslan didn't forewarn us about the progression of the disease, because no one yet knew that people often slid back to psychosis. It would be only two years later, in 2011, when Dr. Dalmau released a paper with a section on that very subject, that the stages of the disease would become widely known.

Lindsey's weekend with me had come to a close. She and our friend Jeff (my karaoke partner in St. Louis), who happened to be in New York for an unrelated trip, were planning to drive the six-teen hours back to St. Louis together. When she called to give him directions, he said he'd like to see me. She warned him I wouldn't be the same.

Jeff rang the doorbell, and my mom invited him inside. He spotted me hovering beneath the staircase, slowly approaching the doorway. He first noticed my smile, a frozen, vacant, idiotic grin that frightened him. I held my arms out, slightly bent, as if pushing my body against a door. Nervously, he smiled and asked, "How are you feeling?"

"Goooooood," I said, drawing out the syllables so much that the one word took several seconds. My lips hardly moved, but I maintained piercingly direct eye contact. He wondered if I was trying to communicate through my stare. It reminded him of a zombie movie.

"Are you happy to be home?"

"Yessssssssss," I said, drawing out the "s" like a strained hiss.

Jeff didn't know what to do next, so he leaned forward and embraced me, whispering in my ear, "Susannah, I want you to know that we're all here for you and thinking of you." I couldn't bend my arms to return the hug.

Lindsey, who stood behind us watching the scene, readied herself for the good-bye. She was not prone to histrionics and hardly ever cried. She had been so stoic throughout the visit, never once letting on how agonizing the stay had been for her, but she couldn't contain herself anymore.

She dropped her luggage on the floor and embraced me. Suddenly I was crying, too.

Lindsey left that morning not knowing if she would ever get her best friend back.

CHAPTER 34

CALIFORNIA DREAMIN'

On April 29, less than two weeks after leaving the hospital, I returned to New York University Medical Center for another week of plasma-exchange treatment. Because my symptoms were no longer considered epileptic but related to autoimmune encephalitis, I was placed on the seventeenth floor: neurology. Unlike the epilepsy unit, this floor in the old Tisch Hospital had not been redone. There were no flat screen televisions, everything seemed dingier, and the patients here seemed older, frailer, and somehow closer to death. A senile woman in a private room at the end of the hall spent her afternoons screaming "PIZZA!" over and over. When my dad asked why, the nurses explained that she loved Fridays, which were pizza days.

I shared a room with an obese black woman named Debra Robinson. Though she suffered from diabetes, the doctors believed that her underlying issues actually stemmed from colon cancer, but they still hadn't confirmed the theory. Debra was so overweight that she was unable to leave her bed and go to the bathroom. Instead, she did her business in a bedpan, periodically filling the room with all sorts of putrid smells. But she apologized every time, and it was impossible to dislike her. Even the nursing staff adored her.

The plasma exchange was done through a catheter inserted directly into my neck. "Oh my god," Stephen said, as he watched the nurse insert the needle. It made a "pop" where it pierced my jugular vein. Holding the catheter in place, the nurse spread heavy tape, the consistency of masking tape, around the catheter to keep it upright, jutting out perpendicularly from the right side of my neck. The tape was so harsh that it left red welts on my skin. Though the catheter was hideously uncomfortable, it had to stay in place for the whole week, over the course of my treatment.

The plasma-exchange process originated with a Swedish dairy cream separator created in the late 1800s that sets apart curds from whey. Scientists were so inspired by this simple machinery that they attempted to use it to separate plasma (the yellow-colored liquid that suspends cells and contains antibodies) from blood (which contains the red and white blood cells). The blood streams into the cell separator, which, like a spin dryer, shakes up the blood, cleaving it into those two components—the plasma and the cells of the blood. Then the machine returns the blood to the body and replaces the original plasma—which is full of the harmful autoantibodies—with a new, protein-rich fluid that does not contain antibodies. Each process takes about three hours. The doctors had prescribed five sessions.

My friends were allowed to come and go as they pleased during this second stay, and they all received specific requests from me: Hannah brought more magazines; my high school friend Jen brought a pumpernickel bagel with butter and tomatoes; and Katie brought Diet Cokes.

On my fourth day in the hospital, Angela arrived for a visit, but she was still startled by how terrible I looked. She later e-mailed Paul that I was "pale, thin, out of it . . . Pretty scary." I still had a long way to go.

It is my last night in the hospital. My roommate Debra just got news: she does have colon cancer, but they caught it early. Debra is celebrating with the nursing staff. They came by to pray with her. I understand her relief, how important it is for your illness to have a name. Not knowing is so much worse. As she prays with the nurses, Debra repeats over and over again, "God is good, God is good."

As I reach to turn out the lights, I feel compelled to say some-
thing to her.
"Debra?"
"Yes, dear?"
"God is good, Debra. God is good."

The next morning I was released again, and Stephen took me
out on a drive in my mom and Allen's car around Summit. We
drove past an old mental institution called Fair Oaks, now a drug
rehab center; the high-school lacrosse field where I once played
goalie; and Area 51, a house on the outskirts of Summit where
our mutual friends lived and partied years ago. When we reached
a red light, Stephen turned on the CD player. The tinkling of Spanish flamenco guitars drifted through the speakers.

"All the leaves are brown and the sky is gray. I've been for a
walk on a winter's day." He recognized the song; it was one of his
favorites, a song that brought him back to his childhood, when
his mother used to listen to the Mamas and the Papas with him
on the way to run errands. "Stopped into a church, I passed along
the way. I got down on my knees and I began to pray."

As if on cue, Stephen and I together belted out the chorus,
"California dreamin' on such a winter's day!" For a moment, Stephen took his eyes off the road and glanced at me in astonishment
and joy. Finally, here was the confirmation he had been waiting
for all these weeks: I was still in there.

IN SEARCH OF LOST TIME

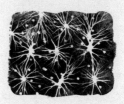

I had only the most rudimentary sense of existence,
*   such as may lurk and flicker in the depths of an*
*   animal's consciousness; I was more destitute of human*
*   qualities than the cave-dweller; but then the memory,*
*   not yet of the place in which I was, but of various other*
*   places where I had lived, and might now very possibly*
*   be, would come like a rope let down from heaven to*
*   draw me up out of the abyss of not-being, from which*
*   I could never have escaped by myself.*

MARCEL PROUST, *Swann's Way: In Search of Lost Time*

CHAPTER 35

THE VIDEOTAPE

I insert a silver DVD marked "Cahalan, Susannah" into my DVD player. The video begins. I see myself at the center of the screen, peering into the camera's lens. The hospital gown slips off my left shoulder and my hair is stringy and dirty.

"Please," I mouth.

On the screen, I stare straight ahead, lying on my back as rigid as a statue, my eyes the only feature betraying the manic fear inside. Then those eyes turn and concentrate on the camera, on me now.

Fear of this sort is not something we typically capture in photographs or videos of ourselves. But there I am, staring into the camera as if I'm looking death in the face. I have never seen myself so unhinged and unguarded before, and it frightens me. The raw panic makes me uncomfortable, but the thing that truly unsettles me is the realization that emotions I once felt so profoundly, so viscerally, have now completely vanished. That petrified person is as foreign to me as a stranger, and it's impossible for me to imagine what it must have been like to *be her*. Without this electronic evidence, I could never have imagined myself capable of such madness and misery.

The video self hides her face under the covers, clutching the blanket so hard her knuckles turn white.

"Please," I see myself plead on video again.

Maybe I can help her.

CHAPTER 36
STUFFED ANIMALS

"What did it feel like to be a different person?" people ask.

It's a question that's impossible to answer with conviction, because, of course, during that dark period, I didn't have any real self-awareness that allowed me the luxury of contemplation, the ability to say, "This is who I am. And this is who I was." Still, my memory does retain a few moments from those weeks right after the hospital. It's the closest I can get to recapturing what it was like to feel so utterly divorced from myself.

A few days after my first hospital stay, Stephen drove me to his sister Rachael's house in Chatham, New Jersey.

I remember the view from the car's passenger seat window, driving past the familiar tree-lined suburban streets. I stared out the window as Stephen's free hand held mine. I think he was as nervous as I was about my reintroduction to the real world.

"Good turkey," I said, out of the blue as we turned into the driveway. It was a simple reference to the night in the hospital when Stephen had brought roasted turkey leftovers for me from his family's Easter dinner. He couldn't help but laugh, and I smiled too, though I'm not certain that I was even in on the joke.

Stephen parked the car next to a woodshed under a basketball hoop. I reached for the door handle, but my fine motor skills were still so weak I couldn't open the car door, so Stephen ran to the passenger side and helped me out safely.

Stephen's sisters, Rachael and Bridget, and their young children, Aiden, Grace, and Audrey, were waiting in the yard. They had heard snippets of what had happened, but most of it had been too painful for Stephen to recount, so they were largely unprepared.

Bridget, for one, was shocked by my state. My hair was unkempt, and the angry red bald spot from the biopsy was exposed, complete with metal staples still suturing my skin together. Yellow crust covered my eyelids. I walked unsteadily, like a sleepwalker with my arms outstretched and stiff and my eyes open but unfocused. At the time, I knew that I was not quite myself, but I had no clue how jolting my altered appearance must have been to those who had known me before. Recalling moments like these, which occurred frequently during this tentative stage in my recovery, I wish I could, like a guardian angel, swoop down and help protect this sad, lost echo of myself.

Bridget told herself not to gawk and tried to hide her nervousness, concerned that I would sense it, but it only made her feel more flustered. Rachael and I had met at her daughter's first birthday party back in October, when I had been outgoing and talkative and, unlike many of Stephen's previous girlfriends, not at all intimidated by the closely knit nature of their family. The transformation was extreme, as though a hummingbird had turned into a sloth.

Because they were toddlers, Audrey and Grace didn't notice that anything was wrong. But Aiden, an outgoing six-year-old, kept his distance from me, clearly unnerved by this strange new Susannah, so unlike the one who had played and joked with him only a few months earlier. (He later told his mom that I reminded him of the mentally handicapped man whom he often saw at their public library. Even in that half state, I could sense his apprehension, though I was bewildered by why he seemed so frightened.)

We all stood in the driveway as Stephen handed out the presents. As soon as I'd gotten out of the hospital, I felt compelled to give away the stuffed animals that had accumulated while I was sick. Grateful as I was for them, they served as plaguing reminders of my childlike state, so I wanted to purge myself of them by handing them off as gifts to the kids. Aiden said a quick thank-you and stood behind his mother as the two girls hugged my leg, each with their own high-pitched "Thank you!"

This initial memory, my first of many interactions with the outside world to come, lasted a mere five minutes. After Stephen handed out the presents, the conversation lulled, as everyone around me struggled internally to keep the superficial flow of words going while also concentrating on ignoring the obvious pink elephant in the room: my shocking state. Would I always be like this? Normally I would have attempted to cover up the silences with my own banter, but today I couldn't. Instead I stood mute and unemotional, internally desperate to escape from this painful reunion.

Stephen was highly attuned to my growing unease, so he put his hand on the small of my back and guided me to the security of the car that would return us to the inner sanctum of our little protected world at home. Though the scene was brief and largely undramatic, and may seem insignificant in the overall scheme of things, it is branded into my mind as a key moment in the initial stage of recovery, viciously pointing out how painful and long the road to full recovery would be.

Another homecoming stands out for me during that same hazy posthospital period: the first time I saw my brother after the hospital. While my life had changed forever, James had been completing his freshman year at the University of Pittsburgh. Though he had begged to visit me, my parents had remained adamant that he complete the year. When school finally ended, my father traveled to Pittsburgh to help bring my brother home, and over the course of the six-hour drive, Dad shared what he could about the past few months.

"Be ready for this, James," my father warned him. "It's shocking, but we need to focus on the positive."

I was out of the house with Stephen when they arrived. My father let James off in the driveway, because my parents, though on far better terms than before, were still not friendly enough for home visits. James watched a Yankees game while he anxiously anticipated my arrival. When he heard the creaking of the back door, he jumped up from the couch.

The image of me walking through the door will remain with him forever, he says. I was wearing oversized, scratched-up glasses, a white cardigan that was two sizes too big, and a mid-length black tent dress that billowed out around me. My face was puffy and unrecognizably distorted. As I wobbled up the steps and through the doorway on Stephen's arm, it seemed as if I had both aged fifty years and lost fifteen, a grotesque hybrid of an elderly woman without her cane and a toddler learning to walk. Even as he watched me, several beats passed before I noticed him in the room.

For me, it was an equally powerful encounter. He had always been my kid brother, but now he had become a man overnight, complete with stubble and broad shoulders. He looked at me with such a devastating mixture of surprise and sympathy that I almost fell to my knees. It wasn't until I saw the look on his face that I realized how sick I still was. Perhaps it was the closeness between us as siblings that brought this realization to the fore, or maybe it was because I had always considered myself an older custodian to baby James, and now the roles were clearly reversed.

As I wavered there in the doorway, James and my mom ran over to embrace me. We all cried and whispered, "I love you."

CHAPTER 37

WILD AT HEART

When I wasn't attending doctors' appointments, my parents allowed me to walk alone to Summit's quaint downtown to get coffee at Starbucks, though they didn't yet sanction solo train trips to visit Stephen in Jersey City. So James mostly drove me around.

It took about a week after James returned from school for him to feel comfortable with this new subdued and disoriented sister. I liked to believe that over the course of our lives, I had played a primary role in James's hipness—sending him Red Hot Chili Peppers CDs at camp, introducing him to Radiohead, giving him tickets to a David Byrne show in Pittsburgh—but now he was the one introducing me to new things. He prattled on about this singer or that movie that we had to see; I had nothing to add.

Despite my being bad company, James spent a lot of his time with me. He worked nights at a nearby restaurant, but when he was free, he would drive me down to the local ice cream parlor for a cup of mint chocolate chip ice cream with chocolate sprinkles, a treat I indulged in at least thirty times during that strange spring and summer. Sometimes we even went twice in one day. We also spent many of our afternoons watching *Friends,* a show that I had never liked before but now became fixated on, though James still disliked it. When I laughed, I would cover my mouth with my hands, but then forget they were there, keeping them by my face for several minutes before mechanically returning them to my sides.

At one point I asked my brother to drive me to town so that I could get a pedicure in preparation for my stepbrother's upcoming wedding. He dropped me off, and I told him that I would call him in an hour, but when my father came to Summit from Brooklyn to check on me and found that I had been gone twice as long without word (I had stopped off for a cup of Starbucks coffee before heading to the salon, which lengthened the trip), he panicked. They frantically canvassed the town, until my father paused in front of Kim's Nail Salon.

He peered into the darkened windows of the spa's storefront and caught sight of me in a massage chair. I looked dazed, staring straight ahead, like I was sleeping with my eyes open. A pool of spit was forming around my lower lip. A few middle-aged women, "Summit moms" as they are called, were throwing uneasy glances in my direction. They seemed to be silently encouraging one another to "check out that crazy girl." My father would later tell me that he was so furious at them he had to move away from the window, prop himself up against the neighboring storefront, and collect himself. After a moment, he took a deep breath and entered the spa with a big smile, his voice booming around the room: "There you are, Susannah. We've been looking all over for you!"

Later the same week, my mom took off work and suggested that we go shoe shopping in Manhattan. As I examined various flats at an Upper East Side store, the salesperson approached my mother.

"Oh, she's so nice and quiet. What a sweet girl," the saleswoman commented cheerfully. It was clear that she thought I was slow.

"She's not *sweet*," my mom hissed, enraged on my behalf. Luckily, I missed the whole exchange.

I fell asleep on my mother's shoulder the way back on the train; the medication and the residual cognitive fatigue from my healing brain made concentrating on acting normal incredibly draining.

Back in Summit, as we headed down the stairs from the train platform, I heard my name. I chose to ignore the voice at first. Not only was I still not quite sure what was real and what was in my head, but the last thing I wanted was to see someone I knew. The second time I heard my name, though, I turned around and saw an old high school friend, Kristy, walking toward us.

"Hi, Kristy," I said. I was trying to make my voice loud and confident, but it came out in a whisper. My mom noticed and spoke for me.

"We were just shopping in the city. We got some shoes," she said, pointing to our bags.

"That's nice," Kristy said, smiling politely. She had heard that I was sick, but had no idea that the problem was with my brain. For all she knew, it had been a broken leg. "How are you?"

I struggled to conjure the loquaciousness that had once been a primary aspect of my personality, but in its place found a deep blankness. My inner life was so jumbled and remote that I couldn't possibly summon up breezy conversation; instead, I found myself focusing on how flushed my face had become and the pool of sweat forming in my armpits. I realized then how great a skill it is to be social.

"Goooooood." I drawled out the word like I had enough marbles in my mouth for a game of mancala. My mind continued to circle around that vast emptiness. *Say something!* I screamed inside, but nothing came. In the silence, I felt the sun beat down on my shoulders. Kristy stared at me with concern. After an awkward moment, she waved her hand and explained that she was running late.

"Well, it was really good seeing you," she offered, turning to leave.

I nodded and watched her glide through the door to the station. I nearly broke down right there in the street. It was amazing how powerless I felt at that moment, especially compared to the superhuman control I had enjoyed during the height of my psychosis. My mom took my hand, realizing the magnitude of this soul-crushing moment, and led me out to the car.

. . .

Despite all this nerve-wracking, zombie-like behavior, James too, like Stephen, saw moments where the "old Susannah" would shine through. Everyone held out hope that I would eventually return. One evening when Hannah came to visit, we sat in the family room watching *Blue Velvet,* a movie by David Lynch, a favorite director of mine. As the first fifteen minutes of the movie played, James and Hannah bantered about its terrible acting. I said nothing, but much later, after they had moved on to a different conversation, I interrupted them to point out, "It's on purpose. The acting. That was David Lynch's style. It's much better in *Wild at Heart.*"

James and Hannah quieted, nodding their heads solemnly. Though they didn't speak about it that night, both would later remember this moment as another confirmation that my old personality was intact, just buried.

CHAPTER 38
FRIENDS

Besides the walks to Starbucks, the *Friends* episodes, and the drives to the ice cream parlor, I spent most of my time in a state of perpetual anticipation as I waited like a puppy for Stephen's arrival on the commuter train to Summit.

Because I couldn't drive, my Mom, Allen, or James had to chauffeur me to the station. One afternoon while my mother and I sat in the car, waiting for him, my mom pointed and said, "There he is! He looks so different!"

"Where?" I said, scanning the crowd. Only when he reached the passenger side window did I finally recognize him: He had shaved his beard and cut his shaggy, cheekbone-length hair into a dapper, slicked-back 1940s hairstyle. He looked even more handsome than usual. As I watched him enter the car, I was suddenly filled with an aching feeling of gratitude that I had found such a selfless, devoted person. It's not as if I hadn't known that all along; it was just that at that very moment, I couldn't contain the deep love I had for him, not only for staying with me, but also for providing me with security and meaning at a very difficult time in my life. I had asked him many times why he stayed, and he always said the same thing: "Because I love you, and I wanted to, and I knew you were in there." No matter how damaged I had been, he had loved me enough to still *see* me somewhere inside.

Though he claims he could see the old me, most other people found it hard to relate. A few days later, I agreed to attend a homecoming party for one of Stephen's and my closest friends, Bryan, who had briefly returned home from Austin, Texas. When we arrived, the grill was going in Bryan's mother's backyard and adults of various ages sat around eating burgers, playing bocce ball, and chatting. As I joined the party with Stephen and his sisters, I felt the air get leeched from the room as everyone seemed to gawk at the sick girl. Though this was likely all in my mind—many of the people had no clue that I had been sick, and even more of them had never met me before—I felt as if I were the center of attention in the worst way.

Yet my friends who were there would later tell me that I seemed unnaturally happy, beaming a plastic and fixed ear-to-ear smile. Maybe that was some sort of self-preserving body armor, a mask to keep the frightening hordes at bay.

At the party, hardly anyone asked me about my hospital stay, though the people who had heard about it approached me diffidently, eyes downcast, seemingly shamed by their knowledge, however slim, of what had befallen me. To these friends, it was like losing me in plain sight while the substitute Susannah was still there to remind them of the person who I had been before. All the while, my mind encircled itself with questions: *Did they hear I was in the hospital? Did they hear I was crazy?* Instead of engaging, I found myself fixedly staring them down, unable to converse. Eventually I gave up trying and concentrated on eating the juicy watermelon and hamburgers cooked on the grill.

But I had my savior: Stephen. People called him the "Susannah whisperer," because he seemed to sense what was unspoken. At the party, he stood by my side, never once letting me stray too far from his watchful gaze. When people who hadn't been debriefed came up to chat with me, he took the reins in the conversation, not something that the normally laid-back, California-cool Stephen did, but something that was now necessary. When I couldn't speak, he spoke for me. Like my plastic smile, Stephen became another layer in my protective armor.

At one point, an old friend, Colleen, who had heard about my hospital stay from Stephen's sister Bridget, noticed that as I ate a piece of watermelon, the red juices dribbled down my chin and onto my dress. She felt conflicted: Tell me or let it be? She didn't want to embarrass me, but she didn't want to let me go on looking like a clueless child. Luckily, before she had to make the decision, Stephen wiped the watermelon juices from my chin.

After an hour at the party, I gave Stephen a look, and he nodded back knowingly. It was time to go.

My second organized social experiment occurred the last week of May at my stepbrother, David's, wedding. I was initially supposed to be a bridesmaid and had purchased the dress just before I got sick, but after I got out of the hospital the bride gently suggested that it might be best if I no longer took part in the ceremony.

Obviously, I thought then, *she's embarrassed by me.*

I realize now that she was acting out of concern, but it was proof to me then that I had become a burden. Normally I was someone people wanted to include—Stephen and I had even been voted "most fun couple" at one wedding we attended prior to my illness—but now I had become a source of shame. This stung and whittled away at my fragile self-worth, which had taken such a thrashing over the prior months.

Still, I was determined to prove to her and the rest of the wedding party that I still "had it." I styled my hair with a straightening iron to cover up my biopsy scar and bought a bubble-gum-pink dress, while Stephen wore a mod-style suit with a skinny tie. A mere month after the reunion at Rachael's house, going to the wedding represented a significant step forward in my recovery process. I was nearly past the period where I looked and acted noticeably awry, though my face was still puffy from the steroids and my words were still faltering and largely monosyllabic. If you didn't look too closely, though, Stephen and I seemed like an ordinary hipster couple.

The ceremony took place in a manor in Hudson Valley, New York, where grapevines dangled along the gates and wildflowers bloomed as far as the eye could see. Stephen and I spent most of the party standing by the makeshift kitchen, where the caterers entered and exited carrying plates of hors d'oeuvres. I don't know if it was the steroids, which can cause an increase in appetite, but I was ravenous.

At the beginning of the night, my mom made me promise that I would drink only one glass of wine. I all but rolled my eyes when I agreed and then went ahead and drank several flutes of champagne. If there's one thing about me that has been confirmed by my illness, it's my tenacity, or bullheadedness, or whatever else you want to call it. Even though my brain was still repairing itself and it's undoubtedly dangerous to mix alcohol with antipsychotics, I insisted on drinking. I didn't care how self-destructive it might be—this was something tangible that connected me to the "normal" Susannah. If the old Susannah had a glass of wine or two with dinner, so would this Susannah. I couldn't read, could hardly make small talk, and couldn't drive a car, but, dammit, I was going to have a few glasses of champagne at a wedding. My mother tried to stop me, but she knew she had no control over my vices: I was going to do what I pleased. Ultimately the wine represented independence, and everyone around me decided it was best not to stamp out what remained of my dignity.

When the song "Build Me Up Buttercup" came on, I even did the twist with Stephen. In my mind, I rocked the dance floor, ignoring the aches and pains in my shins and the fact that I was tiring much more quickly than ever before. (I would later learn from my stepfamily, however, that instead of moving like a pro, I just looked robotic and dazed.)

Despite my attempts at seeming blithe and careless, I was hyperattuned to the different ways people were treating me. Since this was a family event, the first question out of everybody's mouth was, "How are you?" It was an unanswerable question at this stage. But that wasn't the worst part. It was the falsely enthusiastic, carefully enunciated tone people used; they were talking down to me, as if I were a toddler or a very old person. It was demoralizing, but I couldn't really blame them. No one had a clue about what was going on inside my mind.

My mother, however, was proud to see me enjoying myself—that is, until another wedding guest broke into her quiet admiration.

"I'm so sorry to hear what happened to Susannah," the woman said, hugging her. My mother does not like to be touched by strangers.

"Thank you," she said, trying to keep an eye on me.

"It's so sad. She's so different. She's just completely lost her spark." At that, my mom tore her eyes from the dance floor and shot the woman a look. There had been many moments of insensitivity, but this was among the worst. "I mean," the woman continued, "do you think she'll ever get back to her old self again?"

My mom smoothed out her dress, also pink, and shouldered past the woman, saying through clenched teeth, "She's doing very well."

CHAPTER 39

WITHIN NORMAL LIMITS

Although I had already made substantial leaps in my recuperation, nonetheless for many months to come my days would revolve around the candy-colored medications that I had to take six times daily. Each week, my mother spent an hour portioning out my pills into a dispenser that was the size of a shoebox top. Often it took her several tries to get the proportions right because the doses were complicated and always changing. The pillbox was divided into yellow, pink, blue, and green slots and had seven columns for each day of the week and four rows: morning, midafternoon, late afternoon, and bedtime. I was tethered to this pill dispenser.

My reliance on these pills meant I couldn't be independent, and so I loathed them. Not only were they symbols of my infantile status in my mother's home, but the pills also made me sleepy and slow. Sometimes I would just "forget" to take them (an incredibly dangerous thing to do). Because I wasn't wily enough to throw out the medication, I often left the evidence in the dispenser, which tipped off my mother, prompting her to reprimand me as she would a child. In many ways, during that recovery period at my mother's home, I associated the pills—and the fights they engendered—with her. In a practical sense, I needed her to portion out the pills because it was far too complicated a task for me at the time. In a more emotional sense, though, I began to feel that she, like the pills, embodied my contemptible dependence. I can admit now that I was sometimes cruel to her.

"How was your day?" she would ask me after she returned home from a long day at the district's attorney's office.

"Fine," I would say coldly, without elaborating.

"What did you do all day?"

"Not much."

"How are you feeling?"

"Fine."

I cringe when I recall these interactions, since my mom and I had always been inseparable, and I can only imagine how much it must have hurt her. I realize that I was still holding tightly on to an amorphous grudge against her for reasons that seem so merit-less now. Though the hospital was a blur, residual anger from that time remained somewhere in my subconscious. Somehow I had convinced myself that she hadn't spent enough time with me in the hospital, though this was neither fair nor true. On some level, her suffering, which she had buried so deeply, had begun to drain out of her unconsciously and onto me. The worst part was that the struggle didn't end once the hospital stay was over; now she had to live with this hostile stranger, her own daughter, who had once been one of her closest friends. But instead of sympathizing with her pain, which certainly matched and may have even sur-passed my own, I took her suffering as an affront—a sign that she could not handle how flawed the sickness had made me.

She spoke at length about these feelings to Allen but, under-standably, kept them hidden from my father. When my parents spoke to one another, they stuck to discussing how I was doing and hardly engaged in any personal or idle chitchat. Every two weeks, however, they reunited to bring me to Dr. Najjar at his office. Each time he would lower my dosages of steroids; next Dr. Arslan would follow suit with the antipsychotics and antianxiety medications, reducing the amounts in tandem with the changing steroid doses. These were uplifting appointments because each time I seemed to progress steadily, and my parents seemed to be getting along better.

Dr. Arslan would always ask the same question: "Out of 100, what percentage do you feel like yourself?"

Every time I answered with confidence, only my blushing face betraying my inner uncertainty: "Ninety percent." Or, when I was feeling particularly assertive, "Ninety-five percent."

My father always agreed with me, even if he felt differently. But my mom would sometimes gently interject: "I would say more like 80 percent," and this was even a stretch, she would later admit.

Though recovery is clearly a relative process (you need to know where you're coming from to see how far you've gone), we would soon get an expert's view when I attended two evaluation sessions at New York University's Rusk Institute of Rehabilitation Medicine. I was dreading the trip. Although I was clearly getting better, I didn't want proof of my continued inability to accomplish simple tasks. But my mom was adamant that I go.

I recall little from the first session because I was too exhausted to be tested. All I remember are the young psychologist's wide and friendly blue eyes. On the second visit, my mom and dad led me into the Rusk Institute's room 315, where that same psychologist, Hilary Bertisch, led me into her office. My parents stayed in the waiting area. Dr. Bertisch would later tell me that even at this stage I seemed disconnected from my external world and that I often responded to her promptings so slowly that she wondered if I had heard her at all. In some ways, she said, my behaviors resembled the negative symptoms of schizophrenia: inexpressiveness, blankness, lack of feeling, and monotone and monosyllabic speech.

Dr. Bertisch assessed my concentration and memory by providing a letter cancellation test, in which I had to cross out certain words or letters in a normal-length newspaper article, coincidentally enough. She first asked me to cross out all the *h*'s. I got all of them, but it took me 94 seconds, which placed me in the borderline impaired range. Then she had me cross out all the *c*'s and *e*'s. I missed four of these, and the whole thing took me 114 seconds: borderline again. Then came the hardest part: find each use of *and*, *but*, and *the* on the page. I remember feeling confused and constantly forgetting which words to focus on. Out of the 173, I missed 25. Anything more than 15 is considered "severely impaired." My speed, accuracy, and concentration were dismal.

She moved on to working memory, which checks the ability

to hold information in your mind for a short period of time. She read aloud simple mathematical word problems, which were elementary but that I could solve only at the twenty-fifth-percentile range.

My visual working memory was even worse. Dr. Bertisch presented a picture of a shape for a few seconds and then asked me to draw it from memory. No matter how hard I tried, I couldn't imagine the original shape. Here I was in the first percentile, the most severely impaired.

My ability to conjure up words from memory was also fairly poor. Dr. Bertisch repeated the same style of test that had been done in April, when Dr. Chris Morrison asked me to name fruits and vegetables, but this time Dr. Bertisch gave me a minute each to think of as many *f*, *a*, and *s* words as I could:

> F: "Fable, fact, fiction, finger, fat, fantastic, fan, fastidious, fantasy, fart, farm"
> A: "Apple, animal, after, able, an, appeal, antiquity, animosity, after, agile." (Because I had repeated "after" I got only nine.)
> S: "Scratch, stomach, shingle, shit, shunt, sex, sing, song, swim, summer, situation, shut"

Overall, I named 32 words in 3 minutes. Though this was a significant improvement from April, when I could name only 5 words in one minute, the average number of responses is 45.

Yet in other tasks, I had made significant progress. My verbal functioning was now "superior," in the ninety-first percentile. My verbal abstract reasoning, which was tested by using analogies, such as "How are China and Russia related?," was in the high-average eighty-fifth percentile. And despite difficulties with basic cognitive functions, I was still capable of complex analytical thinking, which surprised Dr. Bertisch. On a test involving pattern recognition, I got everything correct, though it took me longer than normal to do so. I couldn't draw an octagon from a visual cue card, but I could make complex leaps in logic. Later she would tell me that the way I presented to people did not match up with what seemed to be going on internally. There was a serious disconnect, and I may have actually been more present than I appeared. I felt this divide too. Often, like at the party and the wedding just a few weeks before, I felt as if my "self" was trying to communicate with the outside world but couldn't break past the broken intermediary, my body.

At the end of our last interview, Dr. Bertisch asked me what I felt were my most pressing problems. "Problems with concentration. With my memory. Finding the right words," I told her.

This she found reassuring. I had defined exactly what was wrong with me. Often those with neurological issues cannot readily identify what is the matter. They don't have the self-awareness to understand that they are ill. Paradoxically my ability to recognize my own weaknesses was a strength.

This explained why social situations were so rough on me: I was aware of how slow and strange I appeared to those around me, especially people who had known me before my illness. I expressed this insecurity to Dr. Bertisch, admitting that I often felt depressed and anxious in groups. She suggested individual and group cognitive rehabilitation, individual psychotherapy to address symptoms of depression and anxiety, and a young adult group.

In the end, though, I was so unsure of myself that I did none of it. In retrospect, this was a big mistake: there is a window of spontaneous healing in the brain after injury or illness, and it's best to jump at any opportunity for faster revitalization. Though it's unclear what role cognitive rehabilitation plays in the recovery from this disease, I would have likely mended more quickly had I done it. But these sessions only highlighted my inner disunity, and I was loath to continue. I never returned for a follow-up. As it was, it took me a year to even decide to track Dr. Bertisch down and get the results of this one group of tests. I didn't yet have the nerve to face how bad off I really was.

CHAPTER 40
UMBRELLA

I couldn't help but consider another hospital stay as a step backward in the march toward recovery, so when Dr. Najjar called my mother in late May to say that I needed to return to the hospital for a second round of IVIG treatment, I was despondent. I shuddered to think of the harsh lights of the hospital room, the constant interruptions of the nursing staff, and those awful preheated dinners. To get my mind off it, my father invited Stephen and me to spend the night, something we did at least once a week now, in his shady backyard, an oasis in the middle of Brooklyn Heights. We ate barbecue, drank sangria, and donned sombreros. A string of multicolored Christmas lights roped around the length of the yard, and Ryan Adams played in the background.

I remained silent for a large portion of the night, as Stephen, Giselle, and my father chatted. Whenever they'd try to include me in a conversation, I shook my head and returned to unconsciously smacking my lips together.

"I'm boring. I don't have anything to say. I'm not interesting anymore," I kept repeating.

"You're anything but boring," my dad would often respond adamantly. It broke my father's heart to hear me say such things. He told me a few years later, in that same backyard and under those same strings of lights, that he would cry himself to sleep thinking of those words.

But no one, not even my father, could convince me otherwise. I was dull, no doubt about it. And being boring was perhaps the toughest adjustment to my new life. This was partially due to the antipsychotics, since the drugs I was on are known to cause drowsiness, confusion, and fatigue. Still, my broken brain itself was likely the most significant cause of my new lack of spirit. It's likely that the electrical impulses between neurons in my frontal lobes were not adequately firing, or they were misfiring and taking longer to get to their intended targets.

The frontal lobes are largely responsible for complex executive functions, prompting experts to refer to it as "the CEO." It only fully develops into our twenties, which tempts many experts to hypothesize that the frontal lobe's maturation is what distinguishes children from adults. But one thing is certain: the frontal lobes make us creative, human, and simply less boring.

(We know, horribly, what happens when the frontal lobe is impaired because of the controversial lobotomy surgeries practiced in the 1950s and 1960s. One such method, the "ice pick" lobotomy, made infamous by Rosemary Kennedy, was a procedure in which a doctor would peel back the patient's eyelid, insert a metal spike above the eyeball until it hit the top of the orbit, and then tap, tap, tap into the brain for several minutes. This imprecise procedure severed several frontal lobe connections, yielding results ranging from dulled emotions to childish behaviors. Some patients were even rendered completely devoid of serious thought and feeling, much like what happened to Randle McMurphy, Jack Nicholson's character in the film *One Flew Over the Cuckoo's Nest*.)

Although my frontal lobes were perhaps taking longer to repair (as some emerging research shows) than other areas, there was nevertheless improvement. In the hospital, one doctor had described my frontal lobe function as being "close to zero." I had, at the very least, improved from nothing.

By the end of dinner, I was so groggy that I put my head on the table and slept straight through the conversation until my own snores woke me up. Shaking myself awake, I headed up the steep metal staircase to the speaker dock that held my iPod. I had recently downloaded the Rihanna song "Umbrella," even though it had been out for a few years and it wasn't even necessarily my typical style of music. Now her stylized, R&B-tinged vocals wafted through the summer night.

I looked down with fondness at my father, Stephen, and Giselle and swayed to the music, suddenly filled with buoyant energy. The music blared, and I began to move my body to the beat, almost absentmindedly, until I was fully rocking out, maybe not exactly gracefully but nowhere near as stiffly and robotically as I had at the wedding a month earlier. Giselle was moved by the glow in Stephen's face when he glanced up and caught me dancing so freely. For a long time it had seemed as if I had existed in a walking coma, but now they all saw life in this awkward reggae dance.

Stephen joined me up on the steps, took me in his arms, and twirled me around, as we laughed at how silly we looked. My father and Giselle joined hands and slow-danced to the upbeat song.

CHAPTER 41

CHRONOLOGY

The brain is radically resilient; it can create new neurons and make new connections through cortical remapping, a process called neurogenesis. Our minds have the incredible capacity to both alter the strength of connections among neurons, essentially rewiring them, and create entirely new pathways. (It makes a computer, which cannot create new hardware when its system crashes, seem fixed and helpless.) This amazing malleability is called neuroplasticity. Like daffodils in the early days of spring, my neurons were resprouting receptors as the winter of the illness ebbed.

It was during that dreaded third hospital stay that my true moment of awakening occurred; I began keeping a diary, started reading again, and first expressed the desire to understand what had happened to me. Perhaps because the diary provides physical evidence of my budding self (I can literally read the thoughts of that wounded Susannah), I can in essence begin to remember what it was like to be her, unlike the earlier Susannah from those paranoid diary entries before the hospital, who was more like a figment of a shadowy memory, so distant that she might have been a character in a horror movie. Yet the person I read about in my recovery diary is childlike and prosaic, unlike that umbral prehospital self who could, even at her most obscured, be eerily illuminating. Yet, there are surprising similarities between this diary and the journals I kept during junior high school. In each, there's a stunning lack of insight and curiosity about myself. In place of deep thought, there are dozens of passages dedicated to my body (weight gain in the recovery piece and lack of breasts in the junior high journal) and silly, petty issues of the day (hating hospital food versus fighting with frenemies). I sympathize with this vulnerable, budding Susannah, as I do that preteen version of myself, but she is still not entirely me, as I am now.

I wrote my first entry at the hospital, dated June 3, 2009, while I was receiving the second IVIG infusion. My father, who had stayed with me every morning as usual during that third hospital stay, helped me write, suggesting that I try to retrace my lost time by compiling a chronology of events from my own memory. My list began with "numbness and sleepiness" and ended with "seizure 3 in the hospital." I had nothing to record after I had bought that cappuccino in the admitting area of the hospital on March 23. In making the list I had also gone back and crammed the words "night at Dad's house" in between "seizure 2" and "seizure 3," almost as an afterthought. This line is the least legible, and with good reason: I was still uncertain and ashamed of my behavior that toxic night (as I am to this day), and it showed even in my handwriting.

My writing was still unfamiliar, but it was a far cry from the infantile notes I had made during my first hospital stay. I could now write in full sentences and even use a semicolon. But what is most telling about my list is the absence: there are no memories at all from my time in the hospital.

My father looked over the page with alarm. It was the first confirmation of my profound memory loss. But he hid his surprise and helped me add in some pieces from his own recollection, providing a more fleshed-out version of events. However, there are still clear omissions, which were both my father's and mine. The gaps are minor but telling, since memory loss can occur not only in brain injury but also with emotional trauma. No one close to me during this time had been spared.

My father indulged in this chronology entirely for my benefit, because he despised speaking of that time. His new motto had become: "To move forward, you have to leave the past behind." But Giselle would later tell me privately how hard the situation had been on him. He was a wreck. When other family members called for updates, he'd wave away the phone, certain that he would lose his hard-won composure once he heard familiar voices. My brother remembers speaking to our dad over the phone while he was still in school and I was still in the grips of a mysterious illness. At one point in the conversation the only sound James could hear on the other line were deep gulps of air meant to mask the sounds of heavy sobs.

Then there is the private journal, which my father, in lieu of talking directly to me about what happened, decided to hand over to me for my research. These entries allowed me to relive the hospital stay from my father's perspective. I read and reread every line; there were moments of laughter and solemn times, and then there were passages so heartwrenching that I wanted to race over to him in Brooklyn and give him a bear hug. But I knew better than to do that. "To move forward, you have to leave the past behind." Though I wasn't ready to do that myself, I could, at least for his sake, follow his motto when it related to him. My strong Irish protector was, at the heart of it all, a big softie, and his love for me, something that during our roughest times I had questioned, was immeasurable. "All I knew was that she was alive, and her spirit was intact. We had more hospital stays for treatments, doctor visits, and lots of medications to deal with, but my baby was on the way home," the journal ends.

Though I never properly thanked my father (or, for that matter my mom, Stephen, my friends, or even the doctors and nurses), we now met for dinner regularly, which was a vast improvement over the once-every–six months relationship we had had before. Sometimes, now, over a meal, we lock eyes and begin speaking in some sort of secret code, which could be described as an otherworldly connection, inadvertently freezing out everyone else at the table. I never realized how rude we often were until Giselle later brought it up. "I don't think you guys are aware of it," she confided, "but sometimes it's hard for people around you to feel included."

We didn't mean to exclude others. My dad and I had gone off to war, fought in the trenches, and against all odds had come out of it alive and intact. There are few other experiences that can bring two people closer than staring death in the face.

. . .

By contrast with my newfound connection with my dad, ever since I was released from the hospital, there had been the cloud of the pills and everything else hanging over my mother and me. I think it's precisely because of how close my mother and I had been prior to my illness that our relationship suffered. Perhaps because my dad had been more of a footnote in my life, whereas my mom was a dominant force, it was easier for my father to engage with this "new" me.

To cope, my mom actively rewrote the narrative of my disease, insisting that I was "never really that bad" and that she "always knew I would recover." I was too strong to be sick forever, she told herself. She couldn't come to terms with the fact that I wasn't yet fully recovered until one afternoon in midsummer when we went out to eat, just the two of us, at J. B. Winberie's in Summit. It was a magnificent evening, with a slight breeze rustling the umbrellas above the patio furniture, so we took seats outdoors and ordered fish entrees and a glass of white wine each.

As we ate, I began to ask her questions about how I had behaved during those days in Summit before I was admitted to the hospital. I still had only nebulous recollections, mostly of things that had turned out to be hallucinations, and I wasn't sure what was real or not. The whole thing was still a mystery to me, and I was eager to piece together what had happened.

"You were just out of your mind," she said. "Do you remember when you had your EEG done?"

EEG? "No, I don't." But after some rehashing, I did remember something: the nurse at Dr. Bailey's office with her strobe light. Unlike the unnerving scene in the hospital video, when my experience of those moments was likely never encoded in my brain at all, this memory had been made and stored. The problem was retrieving it. When the brain is working to remember something, similar patterns of neurons fire as they did during the perception of the original event. These networks are linked, and each time we revisit them, they become stronger and more associated. But they need the proper retrieval cues—words, smells, images—for them to be brought back as memories.

Watching me struggle to remember this, my mom's face flushed, and her lower lip quivered. She buried her face in her hands; it was the first time I had seen her cry since long before I was sick.

"I'm better now, Mom. Don't cry."

"I know, I know. I'm being silly," she said. "Oh, and you were totally nuts. You walked into a restaurant and *demanded* food. Just demanded it. Although I guess that's not too far outside your normal personality."

We laughed. Just for a brief moment, I could picture the rows of booths in the diner and a blurry man behind the countertop handing me coffee. This recovered image taunted me with the echoes of all the other moments I had forgotten and would never get back. And then it was gone.

More than just the recovery of a memory, though, this was the turning point when my mom finally conceded how afraid she had been, revealing through her tears that she hadn't always been certain that I would be "fine." And with that simple, natural gesture, our relationship rounded a corner. She once again became my ultimate confidante, companion, and supporter. It took accepting how close I had come to death (something impossible before, because it was her survival mechanism to deny) to finally allow us to move forward together.

CHAPTER 42
INFINITE JEST

Four months after my initial hospital stay, the lease to my Hell's Kitchen apartment expired. My disability payments, which had been cut in half once they changed from short to long term, could no longer cover the rental expense, so my father met me there one morning to pack up my old life and clear the way for a new, uncertain one.

The red brick tenement was the same as it had always been, with its broken buzzer, stray marks of graffiti, and the "No Trespassing" sign on the door. Piles of unopened mail cluttered my mailbox. The building's superintendent, a chubby, middle-aged man with a thick Spanish accent, walked by us with a short, "How ya doin'?" as if I had never left. Maybe he genuinely hadn't noticed. My father and I climbed the stairs, past the chipping, gray-yellow wallpaper. It was all so familiar that when we made it to my apartment, I half-expected Dusty to still be there waiting for me, even though my friend Ginger had been fostering her for months.

My father and I packed up piles of records, bins of winter clothes, books, pots and pans, and bedding. Halfway through our cleanup, the air conditioner went kaput, which was more than we could bear in Manhattan's blast-furnace July heat. So we returned the next day in the sweltering heat to finally finish the place off.

There is only one line about packing up the apartment in my journal, and it's fairly flippant, like most of my early diary entries: "He helped me pack up my apartment (good-bye living alone)." In this short line, I don't betray the disappointment I felt about having to not only officially abandon my self-sufficient life, but also give up my first real apartment, the symbol of my forgone adulthood. It was one thing to live at my parents' house for a few months, knowing that I had my own place just a train ride away. Now my only home was with my mom; it was like a complete return to childhood. My life of freedom in Manhattan was officially over, at least for now.

The reality was that I was no longer capable of living on my own. It was a fact that I understood but still didn't want to face. Instead I focused on getting my future in order. I began keeping to-do lists with names of people I wanted to thank, projects I wanted to start, or articles I someday wanted to write. Every morning I planned out my day, including insignificant things like "walk to town" or "read the papers," so I could experience the satisfaction of crossing them off. These were crucial little details, because they showed that the frontal lobe, the "CEO," was starting to repair itself.

Instead of attending the cognitive rehab sessions my doctor had recommended, I studied for the Graduate Record Exam, believing for a period of time that school might be the next step in my murky destiny. I bought several study guides to help me prepare, putting every word I didn't know on a flash card, going through them, and then writing down the ones I could not remember. That took up pages and pages of my diary, because I could no longer commit new words to memory as well as I used to.

I also began to read David Foster Wallace's thousand-page dystopian novel *Infinite Jest,* because a pompous professor had once been horrified that I hadn't read it yet. With a dictionary in hand, I read through the novel, stopping every other word or so to find a definition. I kept a running file of all the words that I needed to define from the book. The words I picked are obtuse to me even now, but they are also strangely illuminating:

> *effete* (adj): no longer fertile; having lost character, strength, vitality; marked by weakness or decadence

> *Teratogenic* (adj): of, relating to, or causing developmental malformations

> *Lazarette* (noun): sick room

Despite this studious attention to vocabulary, when people asked me what the book was about I'd have to confess, "I have no idea."

I became preoccupied with my physical state. My diary entries around this time reflect a growing obsession with how much weight I had gained. My distended stomach, cellulite-covered thighs, and bloated cheeks disgusted me, and I tried in vain to avoid my image in any reflective surfaces. Often I would sit outside Starbucks and take stock of the many different types of women walking by: "I'd take her thighs," or "I'd trade bodies with her," or "I wish I had her arms."

I described myself as a "roasted pig," revolted by how my body and face seemed swollen. "Gross," I wrote on June 16. "I make myself sick."

Sure, I had gained a lot of weight since leaving the hospital, where I weighed in at an unnaturally skinny (for me) 110 pounds. Just three months later, I had put on 50 pounds, 20 of which were normal recovery weight and 30 of which were due to side effects of the steroids and antipsychotics, as well as my sedentary lifestyle and constant indulgence in mint chocolate chip ice cream. The steroids also made my face moon-shaped and chipmunk-like, to the point where I hardly recognized myself in the mirror. I had begun to fear that I would never lose the weight and would be forever confined to this foreign body. The problem was much more superficial—but easier to grapple with—than my real worries about being trapped in my broken mind. I know now that I focused on my body because I didn't want to face the cognitive issues, which were much more complex and upsetting than mere numbers on a scale. When I worried about being fat forever, marred in the eyes of those closest to me, I was actually worried about who I was going to be: Will I be as slow, dour, unfunny, and stupid as I now felt for the rest of my life? Will I ever again regain that spark that defines who I am?

The same afternoon as that journal entry, I walked the fifteen minutes from my home to downtown Summit to exert my self-sufficiency and get some exercise. Even though my shins hurt when I walked, I insisted on taking the jaunt to town alone. During my sojourn, a lawn worker stared at me. I instinctively put my hand to my bald spot to shield it from his view, but when my hand touched my head, I realized I was wearing a headband. So what the hell was he looking at? Later it dawned on me: he had been checking me out. Sure, I didn't look my best, but I was still a woman. Momentarily, this boosted whatever was left of my shriveled confidence.

I then decided to take a spin class to address the "roasted pig" syndrome and found myself on a bike next to my high school field hockey coach, who kept looking over, trying to place me. I avoided her gaze, craning my neck to the right, but there I saw two younger girls from high school, also riding bikes. I wondered if they were laughing privately about how fat I was and if they snickered about how I was living with my parents. I felt such shame, but at the time, I couldn't put my finger on the exact reason.

Now, I think that this shame emerged out of the precarious balancing act between fear of loss and acceptance of loss. Yes, I could once again read and write and make to-do lists, but I had lost confidence and a sense of self. Who am I? Am I a person who cowers in fear at the back of a spin class, avoiding everyone's gaze? This uncertainty about who I am, this confusion over where I truly was in the time line of my illness and recovery, was ultimately the deeper source of the shame. A part of my soul believed that I would never be myself, the carefree, confident Susannah, again.

"How are you?" people continued to ask me constantly.

How was I? I didn't even know who "I" was anymore.

After my apartment was packed up and cleared out, I brought home all my unread mail, but I didn't open any of it until a few weeks later. Amid the piles of bills and junk mail, I found a manila envelope sent from the office where I had gotten my first MRI, before I was admitted to the hospital in March. Inside, there was my long-lost gold hematite ring. My lucky ring.

Sometimes, just when we need them, life wraps metaphors up in little bows for us. When you think all is lost, the things you need the most return unexpectedly.

CHAPTER 43

NDMA

As I recovered more and more of my former functions and personality traits, and began to more fully reintegrate myself into the world, I got used to people asking about my rare and fascinating illness. I never tried to articulate it, though, just falling back on the explanation I'd heard my parents repeat so many times: "My body attacked my brain." But when Paul, my editor at the *Post,* wrote asking me to explain the disease to him, I finally decided to try to summarize what had happened to me. This seemed like an assignment in a good way, and for the first time, I felt up to the mission of attempting an answer.

"We want you back!" Paul wrote to me. "God, I sound like Jackson 5. So what exactly do you have?" his e-mail read. It felt strange but also comforting to hear a voice from before my illness: my life was now divided into "pre" and "post" in a way it had never been before. I was determined to get him an answer.

"What is my condition called again?" I yelled to my mom.

"NMDA autoimmune encephalitis," my mom shouted back.

I typed "NDMA" into the search field. An industrial waste product? "What is it again?" I called.

She walked into the kitchen. "NMDA-receptor autoimmune encephalitis."

I Googled the correct term and found a few pages, mostly abstracts of medical journal articles, but no Wikipedia page. After scrolling through several sites, I came across a *New York Times Magazine* "Diagnosis" column on the disease that chronicled the case of a woman who had the same symptoms as I did, but she had the monster tumor, the teratoma. The day after they removed it, she awoke from a coma and started speaking and laughing with family members. The basic explanation about the immune system and the brain was confusing to me. Was this a viral disease? (No.) Was this caused by something environmental? (Maybe, partially.) Is it the kind of disease that you can pass down to your children? (Probably not.) Questions lingered, but I pushed myself to concentrate. I sent Paul a paragraph-long summary of my medical saga, ending, "It's been a crazy couple of months, to say the least. I now know what it's like to go mad."

Paul responded with, "Clears ups a lot of my own curiosity," he said, adding, "And you do realize that your sense of humor and your writing skills have returned, right? I mean that. I can see the evolution in your e-mails and text messages from the time you were sick until now. It's like night and day."

Buoyed by this new ability to explain, I began to research the disease in earnest and became obsessed with understanding how our bodies are capable of such underhanded betrayal. I found, to my frustration, that there's more we don't know about the disease than we do know.

No one knows why certain people, those without teratomas especially, get the disease, and there is no basic understanding of how it is triggered. We don't understand how much impact environment has versus genetic predisposition. Studies seem to point to all autoimmune diseases in general as being about two-thirds environmental, one-third genetic. So did the hypothetical businessman who sneezed on me in the subway really start this horrible chain of reaction? Or was it something else in my environment? I had gone on the birth control patch around the time that my first symptoms cropped up, so could that possibly have instigated the disease? Though Dr. Dalmau and Dr. Najjar have given me no reason to think so, my gynecologist has decided to play it safe and refuses to put me back on the patch. Could my beloved cat have been a trigger? Angela, who later adopted her from me, told me that Dusty had been diagnosed with bowel inflammation, likely caused by an autoimmune disease. Was this a coincidence, or did she and I give each other something that caused both of our immune systems to pounce? Or was there something pernicious lurking around that messy Hell's Kitchen apartment? I will likely never know. But doctors do believe that it was probably a combination of an external trigger, like the sneeze, birth control, or a toxic apartment, and a genetic predisposition toward developing those aggressive antibodies. Unfortunately, since it's so hard to know what causes it, realistically prevention isn't the goal; instead, the focus has to be on early diagnosis and rapid treatment.

Other mysteries prevail. Experts don't even know why certain people have this type of autoantibody, or why it happened to strike during that exact time in my life. They can't say for certain how the antibody gets through the blood-brain barrier, or if it is synthesized in the brain, nor do they understand why some people recover fully while others die or continue to suffer long after the treatment is finished.

But most do survive. And even though it's a hellish experience, the disease is unique in that way, compared to other forms of deadly encephalitis or debilitating autoimmune diseases. It's difficult to find another example where a patient can be comatose and near death, even in an intensive care unit, for many months yet eventually emerge relatively, or even fully, unscathed.

One thing this whole experience is slowly teaching me is how lucky I am. Right time, right place. NYU, Dr. Najjar, Dr. Dalmau. Without these places and people, where would I be? And if I had been struck by this disease just three years earlier, before Dr. Dalmau had identified the antibody, where would I be? Just three years marks the demarcation between a full life and a half-existence in an institution or, even worse, an early ending under the cold, hard tombstone.

CHAPTER 44
PARTIAL RETURN

As he tapered off my dose of steroids, Dr. Najjar prescribed biweekly at-home antibody IVIG treatments once the insurance company finally allowed them to be conducted at home. A nurse would arrive midmornings to hook up my IV to the bags of immunoglobulin over three to four hours. Between July and December, I had twelve infusions.

I continued my correspondence with Paul throughout July. Inevitably every few days he would ask about when I was planning to return to work, and eventually we agreed that the best strategy would be for me to casually stop by the *Post* offices and say hello to the staff without pomp and circumstance. We picked a date in mid-July. I remember the charge I felt as I blow-dried my hair, applied makeup, and plucked my eyebrows, the first time I had done any of that since before I was sick. Then I stood in front of my closet and examined my paltry wardrobe. Only a few things still fit, since I was well ensconced in my "roasted pig" stage, so I chose my trusty black tent dress. My brother drove me to the station, and I took my first independent train ride into the city. From Penn Station I walked uptown to my offices in the scorching midsummer weather.

But when I got to the towering News Corp. building, the place where I had worked since I was a teenager, I felt the rush of adrenaline exit my system, leaving me depleted. *This is too soon*, I realized; *I'm not ready.*

So I texted Paul instead and asked him to meet me behind the building. I had no idea then, but Paul was nearly as nervous as I was, concerned about how I would be in person and how he should treat this new Susannah. Angela, who had visited me recently in Summit, told him that I was significantly improved but still a far cry from the colleague they were used to.

When Paul walked out of the building's revolving door, he saw me and immediately noticed how much I had physically changed: I looked like a little cherub, he thought, like a ten-year-old version of myself, complete with baby fat.

"So how the fuck are you?" Paul asked, hugging me.

"I'm good," I heard myself say. I was so nervous that I could only concentrate on the sweat trickling down my lower back, much like when I ran into Kristy with my mom, but this time I didn't have the buffer of another person to keep the conversation going. It was doubly difficult for me to even focus enough to look him in the eye, let alone prove to him that I would soon be ready to return to work. He cracked some jokes and talked about the job, but I couldn't keep up. I noticed myself laughing at inappropriate times but then missing the cues to his punch lines. I could tell he was trying hard to deflect the awkward silences by maintaining a happy-go-lucky facade, but he was struggling. My state was a bigger shock than he had anticipated.

"I'm still on a lot of drugs," I said offhandedly, hoping to provide an explanation for my changed self. "But by the time I come back, I will be off most of them."

"That's great. We have your desk all ready for you to return. Do you want to come up and say hi to everyone? I know people miss you."

"Nah. I'll do that another day," I said, looking down at the ground. "I'm not ready."

We hugged once more. I watched Paul disappear through the revolving doors.

When he got upstairs, he went straight to Angela's desk. "That's not the Susannah I know," he said.

It was an untenable position. As a friend he was deeply concerned about my recovery and my future, but as a boss, he couldn't help but wonder if I would ever be capable of returning to my duties as a reporter.

...

Nevertheless, two weeks after my brief reunion with Paul, Mackenzie called me up about an assignment for Pulse, the paper's
entertainment section. As I heard her voice, though, it reminded
me of our last interaction: the night in Summit when I had failed
to write the article about Gimp, right around when my seizures
began in earnest. Along with that memory came a sickening feeling of failure. The self-disgust transformed into joy, though, when
I realized she was offering me a new assignment.

"I want you to write about Facebook etiquette," she said.

I may not have been ready to see all my old coworkers, but
I jumped at the opportunity to write an article. I spent a week
manically working on it, treating it like social networking's version of Watergate, calling up sources, friends, and press people to
get their perspectives. But once I put all my notes together in one
file, I stared at the blinking cursor and couldn't picture how to
begin. The memory of that failed Gimp article only intensified my
writer's block. Would I ever be able to write again?

After I sat in front of that blank screen for nearly an hour, though,
the words started to come, slowly at first and then like a fountain.
The writing was rough and needed a lot of editing, but I had put
fingers to keyboard, and nothing in the world felt better than that.

My article ran on July 28 in the *Post*'s Pulse section under the
headline "Inviting Rudeness." I remember making a special trip to
town to pick up the paper that day and glowing with pride when
I opened it and saw my article there. Sure, I'd had hundreds of
pieces published before, but this one mattered more than any other.
I wanted to show the article to everyone, from the Starbucks baris-
tas who had served me coffee all summer, to the younger girls who
rode beside me in that spin class, to the woman at the wedding
who had asked if I would ever regain my spark. This article was my
redemption. It shouted to the world: *I'm back!* That was the most
excited I had ever been about a story running in my whole career. I
wasn't going to graduate school; I was going back to work.

...

And a little over a week later I gathered up the courage to do just that—at least for a brief catch-up. Paul and Angela were out that day, so Mackenzie signed me in downstairs, my ID having long ago vanished somewhere in my hospital blackout. She acted as my chauffeur and protector during the visit. Walking me into the tenth-floor newsroom, Mackenzie felt as if she was dropping a toddler off at her first day of kindergarten. I took a deep breath, smoothed out the same black tent dress that I had worn for my first aborted visit, and headed inside.

No one noticed me. They were too transfixed on the Yankees–Red Sox game. Mackenzie led me past my old desk on our way to Steve's office. "Look who we have here," Mackenzie said to Steve.

Steve looked up from his screen, and it was clear that at first he didn't recognize me. Then he said an uncomfortable but warm hello. "So, when are you coming back?"

My face flushed. "Soon, really soon."

I shifted my weight anxiously from one foot to the next, trying to think of anything to say, but nothing came. When I walked out of his office, my face still flushed by the interaction, a group of reporters who had worked with me on the Sunday paper started to gather. I hadn't talked to most of them for over six months, and though it couldn't have been more than six people, it felt like a mob. I became claustrophobic and sweaty. It was hard to concentrate on any one thing, so I looked at my feet.

Sue, the mother hen of the newsroom, gave me a full-bodied hug. She pulled back and said loud enough for the crowd to hear, "Why are you nervous? We all love you."

The sentiment was kind, but it just made me feel more self-conscious. Was it that obvious that I was uncomfortable? There seemed to be no buffer between what I was feeling and how I appeared. I suddenly felt violently, emotionally naked in front of all these coworkers and friends. I felt like a lab rat, innards exposed, waiting for the impending dissection. The thought jolted me: Would I ever again feel comfortable in this newsroom that basically raised me?

CHAPTER 45
THE FIVE W'S

I did eventually return to work, but not until September, about a month after that partial return and almost seven months to the date after I had my breakdown at work. I recall agreeing obediently as Human Resources suggested that they would start me off slowly at first, part time for only a few days a week. Instead I jumped right back in as if I had never been gone. For years I had pursued my goals like a marathoner: steadily running off to my assignments, jogging to a subway to make it in on time for work, eyes and ears always attuned to the next career step. Now I had had the opportunity to stop, collect my breath, and reassess my destinations, but all I wanted to do was keep on moving.

Luckily the *Post* made it easy for me to dive back in feet first. As Paul had promised, my desk had been left literally untouched: all of my books, documents, and even a paper cup were still sitting there where I had left them.

My first assignments, both briefs, were relatively trivial: one was about a woman voted hottest bartender in New York City and the other a short profile on a drug addict who had just written a memoir. I was being eased back into the daily tasks of writing and reporting, but I didn't care. This fieriness contrasted with my lackluster performance right before I left work seven months before, when I couldn't muster up the verve even to interview John Walsh. Now I met any article, no matter how insignificant, with full and eager enthusiasm.

Though coworkers almost certainly walked on eggshells around me that first month, I didn't notice. I was so focused on the future—on my next byline, on the next assignment—that I couldn't accurately judge what was going on around me. Because I wasn't able to type as quickly as I once did, I recorded most interviews. When I review them now, I hear an unfamiliar voice asking the questions: She speaks slowly and ploddingly, sometimes slurring her words. She sounds tipsy. Angela, my bodyguard, discreetly assisted me with stories without making it seem that I needed the help; Paul would invite me over to his desk as he edited, as if teaching me the five W's of journalism all over again.

It took me over a week to finally get to the task of opening the seven months' worth of unread mail and e-mails. I hated wondering what my sources thought when their e-mails bounced back or were never returned. Did they think I changed careers or moved to a new job? Did they care? These questions plagued me as I trudged through press releases and piles of books.

I was convinced that I was fully back to normal. In fact, I told Dr. Arslan as much when I saw him just before my first week back at work. At that point, I was on such low doses of medication that it was almost negligible. As we did every two weeks, my parents and I sat down around his desk.

"I'll ask you this again. How do you feel out of 100?"

I didn't even hesitate. "100," I replied with conviction. Both my mom and dad nodded their heads this time. My mom finally agreed with my own assessment.

"Well, then, I have to say that you are no longer interesting," Dr. Arslan said with a smile, and with that short statement, he released me from his care. He recommended that I continue on one more week of antianxiety and antipsychotic medications and then stop. I no longer needed them, he explained. To me, this meant that he had made the global evaluation that I had fully returned to health. My mom and dad each embraced me, and afterward we had a quiet celebration over eggs and coffee at a nearby diner.

Although we were in high spirits about Dr. Arslan's appraisal, in reality I still had a long way to go before returning to the person I once was. It's clear now that I was still in the midst of a very imprecise stage in recovery, which Dr. Dalmau and others are studying closely.

"The patients are back to normal, essentially, by family assessments, by friends' assessments, and by physicians' assessments, but they are not back to normal by the same patient's assessment," Dr. Dalmau explained to me during one of our early phone interviews. "And this lingers for quite a long time. Recovery takes as much as two to three years, or even longer."

Patients may be able to return to work, function in society, or even live on their own, but they feel that they have more difficulty doing the things that had once come organically, leaving them essentially still far away from the person they were before the illness.

Right after I returned to work, Dr. Najjar gave me permission to highlight my hair, because the scar, which prevented my hair from growing back as promised, had finally healed enough to stand up to the harsh chemical treatment. I went to the Arrojo salon in SoHo, near the entrance to the Holland Tunnel, where my colorist streaked my hair a bold blond and a stylist cut wispy eye-length bangs that swooped to the right, covering up the bald spot. She asked how I got the scar, so I shared a bit of my story with her. She was so moved that she spent another hour putting my coarse hair (which had changed texture because of the medications) into rollers.

I was feeling like a million dollars as I sauntered down the subway stairway on my way back to Summit until I heard a familiar voice call out my name. I looked around, hoping that I had misheard, to find my ex-boyfriend a few stairs below me. I had not spoken to him since long before my illness.

"I heard what happened," he said sheepishly. "I'm sorry I didn't call, but I didn't think you'd want to hear from me."

I brushed this comment off, we exchanged a few pleasantries, and we said good-bye. This should have been the perfect moment to run into an ex, fresh out of the salon. But it felt destabilizing, and not in a good way. I could tell that he felt sorry for me, and there's nothing worse than seeing pity radiating from the eyes of a former lover.

As I replayed the encounter while I waited on the platform, I caught sight of myself in the oncoming train and noticed how frizzy my curled hair looked, how puffy my face was, and how chubby my frame had become. Would I ever feel comfortable in my own skin again? Or would this self-doubt follow me around forever?

I was nothing like the confident "pre-" person this man had once dated, and I hated myself for how drastically I had changed.

CHAPTER 46

GRAND ROUNDS

Less than a month after I returned to work at the *Post,* my mother received an e-mail from one of Dr. Najjar's assistants, inviting us to attend his lecture on anti-NMDA-receptor auto-immune encephalitis at NYU's grand rounds, the medical school ritual when a doctor presents cases to students and peers.

That late September morning, the commuter traffic was bumper-to-bumper heading from New Jersey into midtown and we were running late. My mom, Allen, Stephen, and I ran to the lecture hall, where my dad, Angela, and Lauren, my friend and the *Post*'s managing editor, were waiting by the entranceway.

"I think it started already," Angela said as we entered the auditorium. The hundred or so seats were filled with white lab coats, all intently watching Dr. Najjar, who was onstage speaking rapidly about "autoimmune encephalitis."

We had missed the introduction of SC, a twenty-four-year-old patient, so I didn't yet realize he was talking about me as he listed all the tests that had come back clean, including three MRIs, hematology and urine toxicology screenings, and blood work. He added that the patient's cerebrospinal fluid had higher-than-normal white lymphocytes, and then discussed his decision to move forward with a brain biopsy when they felt out of other options.

"Is he talking about me?" I asked my parents.

My mom nodded. "I think so."

Dr. Najjar cut to a magnified picture of a biopsied brain sample. It was stained mauve with bluish-purple spots surrounding a blood vessel. The dark spots, he explained, were inflammatory microglia cells.

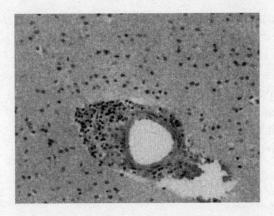

"He's talking about my brain," I whispered, although I didn't understand then what these slides portrayed. All I knew was that a very intimate part of myself was on display in front of a hundred strangers. How many people can say that they've allowed others to literally see inside their heads? I touched my biopsy scar as Dr. Najjar continued to talk about my brain tissue.

He then clicked through to another slide, one that looked like a delicate, chain-link necklace covered with lilac and agate gemstones swooping down in a U shape.

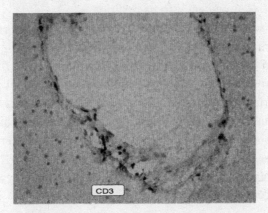

Dr. Najjar explained that the brain biopsy picture showed a blood vessel under attack by lymphocyte cells. As he pointed out, however, there have been only a handful—ten or fewer—of brain biopsies conducted in those with anti-NMDA-receptor encephalitis, so these slides offer a rare and informative look at a sick brain we know very little about.

He ended the lecture with a final statement: "I'm proud to say that this patient is back to normal and is currently back to work at the *New York Post*."

Angela nudged me, Lauren smiled, and Stephen and my parents glowed.

When we got back to the office that day, Angela mentioned the presentation to our editors, Steve and Paul. Steve was intrigued and called me into his office.

"Angela tells me that she went to a meeting on your illness," Steve said. "Would you be willing to write a first-person piece about it?"

I nodded emphatically. I had been hoping my editors would find my story interesting enough for an article, and I was eager to finally indulge my reporting instincts and buckle down to research it.

"Great. Can you get it to us by Friday?"

Today was Tuesday. Friday felt soon, but I was determined to make it happen. It was thrilling, if somewhat frightening and dizzying, to think of sharing those confusing months with the world. Most of my colleagues were still in the dark about what had happened during my extended absence (as, in a sense, was I), and it worried me to think that this story might undo everything I had accomplished in presenting myself as a professional over the past few weeks back at work. But it was irresistible: Now I had the opportunity to uncover that lost time and prove to myself that I could understand what had happened inside my body.

CHAPTER 47

THE EXORCIST

With those conflicting feelings percolating in my mind, I placed my reporter's cap firmly back on and interviewed my family, Stephen, Dr. Dalmau, and Dr. Najjar to get a portrait of my disease and its larger-scale implications.

What I was almost immediately drawn to is perhaps the biggest mystery: How many people throughout history suffered from my disease and others like it but went untreated? This question is made more pressing by the knowledge that even though the disease was discovered in 2007, some doctors I spoke to believe that it's been around at least as long as humanity has.

In the late 1980s, French Canadian pediatric neurologist Dr. Guillaume Sébire noticed an unusual pattern among six children he treated from 1982 to 1990. They all had movement disorders, including involuntary tics or excessive restlessness, cognitive impairments, seizures, normal CT scans, and negative blood work results. The children were diagnosed with "encephalitis of an unknown origin" (or what was colloquially known as the Sébire syndrome), a disease that lasted on average ten months. Four of the six children made what could be called a full recovery. His hazy description of the disease persisted for another two decades.

An earlier paper, written in 1981 by Robert Delong and colleagues, described "acquired reversible autistic syndrome" in children. The disease presented like autism, but two of the three children studied (a five-year-old girl and a seven-year-old boy) recovered fully, while an eleven-year-old girl continued to endure severe memory and cognitive deficits, unable to remember three words provided to her after only a few minutes had elapsed. Now, studies show that roughly 40 percent of patients diagnosed with this disease are children (and this percentage is growing), but children present the disease differently from adults: afflicted children exhibit behaviors such as temper tantrums, mutism, hypersexuality, and violence. One parent described how her child tried to strangle her infant sibling; another heard low grunting noises from their normally angelic daughter; and another child clawed at her own eyes to communicate the inner turmoil that her toddler vocabulary could not convey. The disease in children has often been misdiagnosed as autism, but depending on where and when the person lived, it might have been described as supernatural, even something evil.

Evil. To the untrained eye, anti-NMDA-receptor autoimmune encephalitis can certainly appear malevolent. Afflicted sons and daughters suddenly became possessed, demonic, like creatures out of our most appalling nightmares. Imagine a young girl who, after several days of full-bodied convulsions that sent her flying into the air and off her bed—and after speaking in a strange, deep baritone—contorted her body and crab-walked down the staircase, hissing like a snake and spewing blood.

This chilling scene is, of course, from the unedited version of the blockbuster film *The Exorcist,* and though fictionalized, it depicts many of the same behaviors that children suffering from anti-NMDA-receptor autoimmune encephalitis do. The image is not as exaggerated as we might think. (Stephen, for one, can no longer watch *The Exorcist*; it brings him right back to those strange "panic attacks" I experienced in the hospital, and to my first seizure as we watched TV on the pullout couch.) In 2009, a thirteen-year-old girl from Tennessee displayed a "range of emotions and symptoms that varied by the hour, at times mirroring schizophrenia, and, at other times, autism or cerebral palsy." She lashed out violently and would bite her tongue and mouth. She once insisted on crab-walking across the hospital floor. She also spoke in a bizarre, Cajun-inflected accent, according to the *Chattanooga Times Free Press*, which detailed her experience with anti-NMDA-receptor autoimmune encephalitis and subsequent recovery.

Many parents report that their children start speaking in a garbled foreign language or with an unusual accent, just like when the fictional Regan in *The Exorcist* begins to speak fluent Latin with the priest who has come to exorcise her. Likewise, those who suffer from this type of encephalitis will display what is known as echolalia, the repetition of sounds made by another person. That would explain the sudden ability to "speak in tongues," though in real life those who are suffering from the illness typically do so illogically, not fluently.

How many children throughout history have been "exorcised" and then left to die when they did not improve? How many people currently are in psychiatric wards and nursing homes denied the relatively simple cure of steroids, plasma exchange, IVIG treatment, and, in the worst cases, more intense immunotherapy or chemotherapy? Dr. Najjar estimates that 90 percent of people suffering from this disease during the time when I was treated in 2009 went undiagnosed. Although this number is probably decreasing as the disease becomes better known, there are still people who are suffering from something treatable and not receiving the proper intervention. I couldn't forget how close I had come to such a dangerous edge.

When I contacted her about my research, Dr. Dalmau's colleague Dr. Rita Balice-Gordon brought up the old Indian proverb, often used by neuroscientists studying the brain, about six blind men trying to identify an elephant, offering it as a way of understanding how much more we have to learn about the disease.

Each man grabs hold of a different part of the animal and tries to identify the unnamed object. One man touches the tail and says, "rope"; one touches a leg and says, "pillar"; one feels a trunk and says, "tree"; one feels an ear and says, "fan"; one feels the belly and says, "wall"; the last one feels the tusk and is certain it's a "pipe." (The tale has been told so many times that the outcomes differ widely. In a Buddhist iteration, the men are told they are all correct and rejoice; in another, the men break out in violence when they can't agree.)

Dr. Balice-Gordon has a hopeful interpretation of the analogy:

224 BRAIN ON FIRE

"We're sort of approaching the elephant from the front end and from the back end in the hopes of touching in the middle. We're hoping to paint a detailed enough landscape of the elephant."

Two particular fields of study, schizophrenia and autism, will likely gain the most from this landscaping of the elephant. Dr. Balice-Gordon believes that a percentage, albeit a small one, of those diagnosed with autism and schizophrenia might in fact have an autoimmune disease. Many children ultimately diagnosed with anti-NMDA autoimmune encephalitis were first determined to be autistic. How many children originally diagnosed with autism weren't able to find their autoimmune diagnosis?

As she explained, out of a hypothetical 5 million people diagnosed with autism, 4,999,000 of them might indeed be autistic. But what about that tiny slice that in fact have anti-NMDA-receptor encephalitis or one of the other related disorders, and could be effectively treated by looking for a peripheral tumor or antibodies in the brain?

The same goes for schizophrenia. Many of the adults ultimately diagnosed with anti-NMDA-receptor autoimmune encephalitis first receive the diagnosis of schizophrenia (or other related mental disorders, such as schizoaffective disorder, in my case). Statistically there must be some people who receive a diagnosis of psychosis or schizophrenia and never get the proper help. Even if it's only 0.01 percent of patients, it's still too many.

Unfortunately, for most people suffering from severe psychiatric conditions, it's nearly impossible to give everyone the proper testing to diagnose and treat autoimmune diseases. PET scans, CT scans, MRIs, IVIG treatment, and plasmapheresis can cost upwards of thousands of dollars each.

"How practical would this screening be?" asks professor of psychology Philip Harvey. "Lumbar punctures for everyone? That's an impossibility."

It had cost $1 million to treat me, a number that boggles the mind. Luckily, at the time I was a full-time employee at the *Post*, and my insurance covered most of the exorbitant price tag. I also had a support system in place. My family was in the fortunate situation of being able to pay out of pocket anything that the insurance company wouldn't cover or reimburse. Unfortunately, there's often not the same safety net in place for those with life-long psychiatric conditions, who are unable to hold jobs and must make do with disability payments and Medicaid.

But this is all the more reason that psychiatrists and neurologists are finding ways to break down the barriers set in place between psychology and neurology, urging for one uniform look at mental illnesses as the neurochemical diseases that they are, and, in the process, perhaps getting more grant money to study the overlap.

"One thought is that this is just a coincidence, that [NMDA-receptor encephalitis] and schizophrenia are unrelated. But Mother Nature doesn't work that way. The best hypothesis for schizophrenia is that at least some of those cases can also be explained by a [similar] dysfunction," said Dr. Balice-Gordon.

Dr. Najjar, for one, is taking the link between autoimmune diseases and mental illnesses one step further: through his cutting-edge research, he posits that some forms of schizophrenia, bipolar disorder, obsessive-compulsive disorder, and depression are actually caused by inflammatory conditions in the brain.

Dr. Najjar is in the midst of groundbreaking work that might finally sever the barrier separating immunology, neurology, and psychiatry. A recent case of his centers on a nineteen-year-old woman who had been diagnosed with schizophrenia by six leading psychiatrists over the course of two years. When she was seventeen, her symptoms began with auditory hallucinations—"people putting me down and thinking they're better than I am," she told Dr. Najjar—followed by visual ones. Late at night, she would see "people's faces on the walls."

Her parents did not believe the schizophrenia diagnosis and eventually made their way to New York University, where they met with Dr. Najjar. He ordered a right frontal brain biopsy—

something he had learned from my case—that showed the presence of inflammation and antibodies targeting the glutamate
receptors in the brain. She was treated with steroids, plasma
exchange, and IVIG treatment, which helped with the hallucinations and paranoia, but because the treatment was started so late,
it is unclear if she ever will return to her former self.

"Just because it seems like schizophrenia doesn't mean that it
is," Dr. Najjar told me. "We have to keep humble and keep our
eyes open."

As I researched my article, I was curious to get the perspective of Dr. Bailey, the neurologist who had asserted that my problems stemmed from alcohol withdrawal and stress, to see what
he thought about the ultimate diagnosis. When I reached him by
phone, though, it turned out he still had never heard of the illness,
even though my diagnosis had been discussed in almost every
major medical journal, including the *New England Journal of
Medicine,* and the *New York Times.*

In the spring of 2009, I was the 217th person ever to be diagnosed with anti-NMDA-receptor autoimmune encephalitis. Just
a year later, that figure had doubled. Now the number is in the
thousands. Yet Dr. Bailey, considered one of the best neurologists
in the country, had never heard of it. When we live in a time
when the rate of misdiagnoses in the United States has shown no
improvement since the 1930s, the lesson here is that it's important
to always get a second opinion.

While he may be an excellent doctor in many respects, Dr. Bailey is also, in some ways, a perfect example of what is wrong with
medicine. I was just a number to him (and if he saw thirty-five
patients a day, as he told me, that means I was one of a very large
number). He is a by-product of a defective system that forces neurologists to spend five minutes with X number of patients a day
to maintain their bottom line. It's a bad system. Dr. Bailey is not
the exception to the rule. He is the rule.

I'm the one who is an exception. I'm the one who is lucky. I
did not slip through a system that is designed to miss cases just
like my own—cases that require time and patience and individu-

alized attention. Sure, when I talked to him, I was shocked that he knew nothing about the disease, but that wasn't the really shocking part; I realize now that my survival, my recovery—my ability to write this book—is the shocking part.

Yet even after all of this, the most harrowing part of researching and writing the article about my illness was something that I had in no way prepared for: handing over the EEG tapes to my paper's photo editor, who wanted to use some images of me in the hospital for the piece. I hadn't yet watched them and at that point did not plan to.

But when he had trouble opening up the disk, he asked me for help. I got it to work and in the process caught a fleeting glimpse of myself in the hospital gown. I was outrageously skinny. Crazed. Angry. Reaching out aggressively toward the camera.

I shuddered and turned away from the image, trying to concentrate on breathing as I forced a smile. I had the intense urge to grab the videos from him and burn them or at least hide them away, safe from view. Even after everything I'd done and learned, maybe I wasn't ready for this yet. Yet I felt compelled to keep watching.

I had enough distance from my own madness to view it as a hypothetical. But watching myself on screen, up close and personal, obliterated that journalistic distance. The girl in the video is a reminder about how fragile our hold on sanity and health is and how much we are at the utter whim of our Brutus bodies, which will inevitably, one day, turn on us for good. I am a prisoner, as we all are. And with that realization comes an aching sense of vulnerability.

That night I went home and passed a night of fitful dreams that blurred together. In one, I was with my mom and Allen in Summit.

"Remember when you were in the hospital," my mom said, laughing really hard. "You were so crazy that . . ."

She was laughing so hard that she couldn't complete the sentence.

"What happened?" I asked, grabbing a notebook and a tape recorder. She was laughing, gulping in air, too hysterical to talk, still laughing.

There was a second dream that blurred together with this first one. In it, I was on the epilepsy floor, but I was completely naked and in search of a bathroom to hide in. I heard a group of nurses walk by and tried to hide, but as I turned the corner, all of a sudden I saw Adeline, the Filipino nurse from the floor. Now I was fully clothed.

"Susannah," she said. "I hear you're not taking care of yourself. What a shame."

Though I hesitate to draw any Freudian meanings from these dreams, they clearly represent the anxiety I felt about how I behaved in the hospital and how others perceived me during my recovery. This was not where I wanted to be psychologically as I started working on my first major assignment back at the *Post*. I didn't want to be frazzled and upset, and these tapes had obviously upset my internal balance.

But, ready or not, on Sunday, October 4, the biggest story of my career ran in the *Post* under the headline: "My Mysterious Lost Month of Madness: I was a happy 24-year-old suddenly stricken by paranoia and seizures. Was I going crazy?"

CHAPTER 48
SURVIVOR'S GUILT

It is one thing to research your own condition and think abstractly about the other people who have suffered from the same condition; it's another thing entirely to get to know the people themselves who have run the risk of being lost in the system.

Because I had been the only person ever to be diagnosed with anti-NMDA-receptor autoimmune encephalitis at NYU, I had felt as if I was in a rarified group of the walking wounded without any compatriots with whom to share war stories. I was wrong.

Although anti-NMDA-receptor autoimmune encephalitis is rare, it is one of the more than one hundred different kinds of autoimmune diseases that afflict an estimated 50 million people in the United States, a staggering figure that has more than tripled in the past three decades. An alarming majority of autoimmune diseases—around 75 percent—occur in women, affecting us more than all types of cancer combined. Autoimmune diseases are most likely the number one cause of disability in women of all ages. There are multiple theories about why women are so disproportionally affected, ranging from genetic, to environmental, to hormonal (most women are of childbearing age when they are diagnosed), to the fact that women's immune systems are more complicated (they need to identify and safeguard fetuses, which are half-foreign entities, during pregnancy), and with everything more complex, malfunctions are all the more severe. For now, it's just one more riddle in a series of question marks.

Dr. Dalmau and his lab have also identified other receptor-seeking autoimmune diseases that occur in the brain, making the anti-NMDA-receptor variety still rare but not unique. Now antibody-mediated autoimmune diseases have become a bona-fide group of syndromes. Dr. Dalmau's lab has identified six other types of antibodies that target various receptors in the brain, adding to the NMDA-receptor-preying kind, which struck me. This figure is growing. Dr. Dalmau estimates that when all is said and done, there could be twenty or more. These discoveries finally will give names to diseases vaguely referred to as "encephalitis of an unknown origin," or "psychosis not otherwise specified," or not given any designation at all.

So it was no wonder that after the *Post* article ran, my inbox filled with hundreds of e-mails from mothers and fathers whose children had recently been diagnosed with all kinds of autoimmune diseases, women my age in the throes of the same disease, and people who suspected that their loved ones had it and wanted information on how best to treat it. Like any other major trauma, this disease bursts you wide open, and after surviving so much, you're finally prepared to give back and willing to help anyone else who may be going through similar upheavals. But being so exposed, like a gushing wound, leaves you unprotected from the elements.

Many of the stories that I heard from that time were similar to my own, if not more harrowing. The words of people I spoke with kept me up at night: *Why me? Why did my antibodies decide to attack? Why was I able to then recover?*

I live with that constant refrain—not of self-pity but the real question of why my body decided to turn on itself. Then again, why does this happen to anyone? There are now thousands of cases of anti-NMDA receptor autoimmune encephalitis and many that have not ended well: an elderly woman who passed away because she had been misdiagnosed with a urinary tract infection; a woman who was pregnant when her symptoms progressed had lost her baby; several girls who had their ovaries removed when the doctors could not find a teratoma and the immune suppressants that had worked wonders on me didn't help them.

Almost everyone I spoke to had experienced delusions and hallucinations: a music teacher saw and heard a full symphony outside her window; a young woman called out for a priest, requesting an exorcism because she was certain she was inhabited by the devil; another woman my age hated herself so much during her recovery that she ripped out her hair and cut her arms. Paranoia, especially about the men in their lives, was also a common thread. A middle-aged woman believed that her husband had fathered a baby with a neighbor; a young teenager was convinced that her dad was cheating on her mother. One twelve-year-old I spoke to tried to jump out of a moving car; another woman had an obsession with grapes (like my fixation on apples).

All the people I spoke to had lost themselves. And not everyone had found herself again. Some would never be as smart or funny or animated as before the illness.

There were even calls from people who had been diagnosed with schizophrenia and were desperate for any other answer. My story gave them hope, but some of these people scared me with their persistent paranoid phone calls.

"You know they're listening to us," one older woman said.

"I'm sorry?"

"They're bugging my line. So I can't say much."

"I hear voices," another person said. "There are people out to get me. Just like you."

One woman who sounded manic, her pressured speech hard to understand, called several times a day, trying to arrange a meeting so that I could diagnose her myself.

"I'm not a doctor, but you should contact these people," I said, providing these callers with the list of doctors who had treated me. But the truth was, the only difference between those suffering from schizophrenia and me was that I was cured. Like these people, I knew exactly what it was like to be caught in the prism of your own fractured psyche.

Survivor's guilt as a kind of posttraumatic stress disorder (PTSD) is common—a study indicates that 20 to 30 percent of survivors develop it—and it has been documented in those with cancer and AIDS, as well as war veterans. I can sincerely relate to this feeling, even though in some ways, my problem is the opposite of PTSD: whereas most PTSD sufferers are desperately trying to escape their memories of the original trauma, I have none.

But still the guilt remains, especially when I speak to families who cannot help but feel resentful. There was a newlywed who called me about his wife; he had e-mailed me on Facebook, and I gave him my number. "How do you know you won't get sick again?" he asked, aggressively.

"I don't know. I really can't answer that."

"How can you be sure?"

"I can't be. This is just what the doctors are telling me."

"And how come you got better while my wife is still sick, even though she was diagnosed before you?"

"I, I don't know."

Two weeks later, he called me back. "She's dead. She died last week. I thought you should know."

There had been no miracle diagnosis for his wife. And there is not a miracle diagnosis for everyone. There doesn't seem to be any logic to it; it's the luck of the draw, as unfair and callous and, frankly, terrifying as that may sound. Even if the disease is properly treated, there is still about a 25 percent chance that someone with it will be permanently disabled or die.

But there are many more interactions that I've had in the wake of this illness that have turned this terrible disease into some sort of gift—not one that I would bestow even on my worst enemy but a gift nonetheless.

I became close to a woman named Nesrin Shaheen, whose preteen daughter developed the illness around the time that I did and now works tirelessly to spread awareness, devoting countless hours to a Facebook page on anti-NMDA receptor encephalitis that helps hundreds of people navigate the lonely illness. In addition to Nesrin's Facebook page, many other sites are devoted to spreading the word and connecting patients and families so that they don't have to go through this ordeal alone.

. . .

The most affirming moment of my entire life—and to be able to say this with absolute certainty is just another example of how this disease has changed my perspective in positive ways—was when a man named Bill Gavigan called me in spring 2010.

"Is this Susannah Cahalan?" he asked breathlessly.

"Yes," I said, taken aback. People usually did not say my name as if it carried such weight. He went on to tell me the story of his teenage daughter, Emily.

One day when she was a sophomore at a Pennsylvania college, Emily suddenly started speaking rapidly and became paranoid that pickup trucks were following her, communicating her whereabouts to each other on walkie-talkies. The next day, when they were headed to a Broadway show in New York, Emily became fixated on the cars around them. She insisted that they were being tailed, which so worried Bill and his wife, Grace, that they immediately turned the car around and headed straight to the ER. In the hospital, Emily's paranoia intensified because the ER doctor reminded her of her high school history teacher, which convinced her that he was an imposter, an actor playing the part of a doctor—exactly what had happened to me with my father and the EEG nurse.

Emily admitted herself into a psychiatric ward, where she stayed on observation without any contact with her family for seventy-two hours. She was put on a litany of mood stabilizers and antipsychotics and remained in the ward for another two weeks before she was released with the diagnosis of "psychosis, not otherwise specified," medical jargon for "we have no clue."

Although she was heavily sedated, she insisted on returning to school. But then her parents received a call from the dean of students, expressing grave concern over Emily's erratic behavior. She returned home, and for the next few weeks was shuffled back and forth between her parents' house and the local psychiatrist, until she was admitted to the Psychiatric Institute of Pennsylvania for three weeks. Bill compared the experience to the movie *One Flew Over the Cuckoo's Nest.* Though they did not have a diagnosis yet, the psychiatrist told her parents that he was leaning toward schizophrenia, even after other neurologists had offered a possible diagnosis of multiple sclerosis. The social worker there advised them to sign her up for social security disability because "she's never going to be able to work." Bill refused to believe that and threw the social security forms in the trash after she left.

It was around this time that Bill's sister, Mary, saw me on the *Today* show (after a producer who saw the *Post* piece invited me on for a segment). She sent the video to Bill, who passed it and my *Post* article along to Emily's psychiatrist.

"She didn't have seizures," said the psychiatrist, pointing out the discrepancies between my case and Emily's. He seemed genuinely insulted by the implication that he had missed something. "You have to come to terms with the fact that you have a daughter with mental illness."

After twenty-one days at the institute, Emily went through outpatient treatment and eventually returned to school yet again, completing the semester with good grades even though her parents still believed she wasn't 100 percent well.

It appeared that she had overcome the problem, whatever it had been, until she came home for spring break, when her physical and cognitive issues suddenly got dangerously severe. Bill noticed that she could no longer solve simple math problems; Grace watched her daughter try to eat a pint of ice cream, almost unable to hold her spoon. Then, suddenly, she went from speaking too fast to not speaking altogether.

She was rushed to the nearby hospital, where the doctors informed Emily's parents that an MRI from a year ago had shown inflammation, a fact that had never been shared with the Gavigans before. As the doctors prepared for an aggressive treatment of IVIG, which helps with inflammation, Emily developed a blood clot in her brain, which caused her to seize for an hour and a half.

While Emily was convulsing in the next room, Bill thrust my article into the on-call neurologist's hands.

"Read this. Now," he commanded.

The doctor read through it right in front of Bill, placed it in his pocket, and agreed to test her for this rare autoimmune disease.

As soon as she could be moved, Emily was air-evacuated to the University of Pennsylvania, where Dr. Dalmau's colleagues diagnosed her and began treatment for anti-NMDA-receptor encephalitis. Through an aggressive regimen of steroids and chemotherapy, Emily has returned full time to college. She is 100 percent healthy now and in 2012 finished her final semester of college.

On the phone to me, her father said, "I don't want to be, well, I guess there's no way other than to be very dramatic about it. But I'm not kidding, if we didn't have that article to hand to the doctor, she'd be dead."

He also sent me video footage of her skating with a note: "I thought you might like to see Emily skating. This is the first time I have seen her skate in two years. She is in the middle of the ice when the video starts. Also, as we were reflecting this past weekend since it was Mother's Day, I remembered taking her in a wheelchair last Mother's Day to the gift shop in the hospital to buy her mother a card, and she was unable to speak or walk. A year later, she is able to ice skate like you will see in this video. We continue to count our blessings."

I clicked open the cell phone video and watched her. Emily wears a pink skirt, black leggings, and a black shirt, with a pink ribbon tied in her hair. She's so natural on the ice that she seems to float just above its surface as she pirouettes, spinning and spinning in the center of the rink.

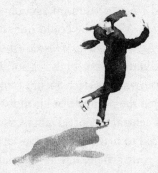

CHAPTER 49
HOMETOWN BOY MAKES GOOD

The *Post*'s "Month of Madness" article changed not only my life but Dr. Najjar's as well. After its publication, Dr. Najjar invited me to his house in Short Hills, New Jersey, about a five-minute drive from my mom's Summit home. He answered the door and introduced me to his three teenage children and his wife, Marwa, a lovely woman with fair skin and light hair, several years younger than her husband. They met at the New York Infirmary Beekman Downtown Hospital (now part of NYU) in 1989, where he studied neuropathology and she worked in the lab. One afternoon, the shy Souhel made a joke in Arabic, and to his surprise, she laughed. She didn't look Middle Eastern, but when he introduced himself, he found that she too came from Syria.

Marwa offered me tea as we sat in their living room by a grand piano. Midway through the conversation, Dr. Najjar mentioned his father, Salim Najjar, and seemed proud to share his incredible story.

Salim had grown up in an orphanage. His mother, who worked long hours at a nearby hospital making lab coats for doctors (coincidentally), had to give Salim up as a child when his father suddenly passed away. Alone, she could not support him on her meager income. Salim, who had so stressed education for his own sons, had never graduated from high school, but through sheer will and a tendency toward perfectionism, took up the construction trade and reached the pinnacle of his industry when his company built the city's central airport, Damascus International. But none of this compared to his son's successes overseas.

"My father saw your article. It was translated into Arabic in multiple papers. Not just one," Dr. Najjar said. "There were, I mean, tears."

"No way," I said.

"Yeah, he had it framed and everything."

After my article ran, the Syrian ambassador to the United Nations had reached out to Dr. Najjar to congratulate him on a job well done and then sent my *Post* article to SANSA, a Syrian news agency. Overnight, every news outlet there covered the story of how a Syrian boy had become a miracle doctor in America.

"Remember, this is the dunce. The class dunce who couldn't do the work." Marwa smiled. "The hometown boy makes good. You made it, baby, way to go."

Later that same year, Dr. Najjar was named one of *New York Magazine*'s best neurologists in the country.

CHAPTER 50
ECSTATIC

By the time the *Post* published my piece, most people who knew me would have agreed, "Susannah is back." I had returned to the *Post* full time, Dr. Najjar and Dr. Arslan had finally taken me off all medications, and I had even navigated the treacherous waters of live television in early 2010 when I was a guest on the *Today* show to discuss my illness.

Since my mom and Allen had decided to sell their Summit house, Stephen and I moved in with each other far sooner than either of us had anticipated. We both skirted the issue for months as I scrolled through ads looking for a studio apartment that would fit my tight budget. After a few weeks of searching, it became clear that I couldn't afford to live alone. I dreaded bringing up the option to live together for fear that I would be pushing him to that next relationship step too soon. And I felt it wasn't fair to press him: How could he say no? But when I impassively broached the subject with him he said, without hesitation, "That's what I assumed we'd be doing."

Still, Stephen was privately anxious about taking on the role of caregiver, despite how well I was doing. If something happened to me under our shared roof, he would be responsible. But he decided to press on: I was too broken, financially, emotionally, and physically, to live alone, and he wouldn't have wanted us to be separated anyway.

So now you could add the grown-up step of living with my boyfriend to the list of reasons showing that I was "back." But in reality it took several more months for me to assuredly say that I felt comfortable in my own skin again, when I finally could rely on myself not to wince when I ran into ex-boyfriends or cower in the back of a spin class.

This eureka moment happened quietly, more than a year after my diagnosis, when I was visiting my extended family in Santa Fe, New Mexico, for my cousin Blythe's wedding in June 2010. At that wedding, unlike the one I had attended early in my recovery, there was no longer a chasm between the person I was inside and what people around me saw. I felt in control and at ease; I no longer struggled for the right words, didn't have to push myself to make small talk, and had reclaimed my old sense of humor.

Because they had almost had to mourn me, friends and family feel relatively comfortable speaking openly about their relationships with and impressions of me. Because of this, I often felt like Tom Sawyer attending his own funeral; it's a strange kind of gift. Two words keep repeating: *outgoing* and *talkative*. Almost every single person uses some variation of those words to describe me. I had never really known how much these terms had defined me and how jarring it must have been when I had suddenly become neither of those things.

I know that this new Susannah is a lot like the old Susannah. There are changes, but it's more like a step to the left than an overhaul of my being. I talk fast again, can do my job with ease, feel comfortable in my own skin, and recognize myself in pictures. However, when I look at photographs taken of me "post," versus pictures of me "pre," there is something altered, something lost— or gained, I can't tell—when I look into my eyes.

But recognizing myself in pictures, of course, does not signify a full return; I'm different than I was before. When I try to pinpoint all the subtle ways that I have changed, my hand instinctively sneaks up to that raw, bumpy bald spot on the front of my scalp that will never grow hair again. It is my permanent reminder that no matter how "normal" I feel, I will never be the same person that I was before.

However, there are far scarier things that concern me about this new Susannah. I talk in my sleep every night, something that I did not do before. One night, Stephen woke up to my screaming, "There's a container of milk over there. A huge container of milk!"

In a way, it's funny, but given our experiences, also slightly sinister. And I have fears now that the carefree pre-illness Susannah did not have. A few months ago, a concerned parent called to update me about his daughter, who had relapsed. He shared another story about a woman who had made a full recovery for several years but recently had been stricken with the disease again while traveling abroad. Apparently relapses happen in about 20 percent of cases. Unlike cancer, there is no remission date. After a full recovery, you could relapse tomorrow as easily as five years from now. Those who did not have a teratoma, like me, have a higher rate of relapse, for reasons unknown, but at least those who do relapse tend to have the same rate of recovery as they did after the initial onset of the disease. This does little to ease my mind.

Recently, as Stephen and I were watching TV in our Jersey City apartment, out of the corner of my eye I saw something move on the floor.

"Did you see that?" I asked Stephen.

"See what?"

"Nothing." *Am I going crazy again? Is this how it's going to happen?*

Then I saw it again. This time, Stephen grabbed his shoe and squashed the two-inch-long water bug.

I live with this fear. It does not control me or hinder my resolve, but I do live with it. The friends and relatives I interviewed would never have used the term *skittish* to describe me, but every now and then, when I'm on the subway and the colors seem brighter than normal, I think, *Is it the lighting, or am I going crazy again?*

And what about the subtler changes that cannot be touched or easily identified? I asked Stephen if he thought I was different now. Am I suffering from cognitive defects of which I am unaware? After a moment, he shook his head, "No, I don't think so." But he seemed uncertain.

Those closest to me had undoubtedly changed as I did, if not even more so. Stephen, who was once always so laid back, had become a worrier, especially when it came to me.

"Do you have your phone? How long will you be gone? Call

me the minute you leave," he would often repeat, calling and texting me over and over if I went just a few minutes without answering my phone.

For a long time after the hospital, Stephen saw me as a piece of fine and fragile china that could easily break, and he continued as my protector against the cracks and fissures of the real world. Though I'm eternally grateful for this, sometimes it became exasperating when he couldn't give up that role. How could you blame him? But I did. Accepting this type of nannying was completely outside my personality, normally so self-reliant and obtusely independent. So, perversely, I would battle him, staying out late without calling and pushing his buttons about his constant check-ins. It was only when I started acting like an adult that Stephen started to treat me like one, and slowly we became equals again, evolving into a healthy relationship so different from the caregiver-patient relationship that had been formed under the harsh lights of the hospital room. But of course he still worries, and I doubt this will ever change. His thoughts often return to that night at my Hell's Kitchen apartment, where my eyes rolled back in my head and my body stiffened, and both of our lives changed forever.

Yet some things haven't changed. My parents, who had briefly been able to put aside their deep-seated animosity during my hospital stay, weren't able to maintain their civil relationship after I had returned to myself. Without doctor appointments keeping them in contact, they fell back into the routine of habitual avoidance that even their daughter's near-death experience couldn't mend.

People never change, they say. I remember when I was entering sixth grade and the guidance counselor called us into her office to talk about the transition from elementary school to middle school. She asked me to pick an emoticon out of a list of about fifty to describe how I felt on the first day of school. I picked "ecstatic," the one with the wide-mouthed, full laugh. The counselor was surprised by my pick; this apparently was not a common choice. I had been ecstatic then, but would I pick ecstatic now? Or have I lost that spark after all? Is there a sliver of me that did not recover from the fire?

CHAPTER 51

FLIGHT RISK?

The impostor EEG nurse, the sea of paparazzi surrounding my father at the top of the news hour, the insult silently hurled at me by my stepfather. These absurd memories persist, while others that are real and documented fall through the fingers of my mind like water. If all I remember are hallucinations, how can I rely on my own mind?

To this day, I struggle with distinguishing fact from fiction. I even asked my mother if Allen had actually called me a slut in the car that day.

"Are you kidding?" my mom asked, hurt that I could even ask. "He would never do that."

She was right; logically, I understood he would never say such things. Yet why did I continue to believe my own bizarre memory over a lifetime of proof? And why did these specific memories remain intact? If I didn't have a mental illness, how did these hallucinations come about?

Though hallucinations, paranoia, and an illusory grasp on reality are the hallmarks of those with schizophrenia, you don't need to suffer from a mental illness to induce these symptoms. In 2010, a Cambridge University study helped to illuminate the thought processes of people with schizophrenia by injecting healthy student volunteers with the drug ketamine—which blocks the same NMDA receptors in the brain that were affected by my illness—and conducting what is known as the "rubber hand illusion" on them. Fifteen students were asked to place one hand on a table beside a fake rubber hand, first after they had been injected with ketamine and then at a later sitting with a placebo. During the experiment, the real hand was hidden from view as two paint-brushes, attached to motors, stroked the index fingers of both hands. Though subjects on a placebo could also be tricked by the illusion, those on ketamine sooner and more intensely believed that the rubber hand was their own. The experiment showed that the ketamine injections, for whatever reason, helped break down the subjects' sense of reality, making things that would ordinarily seem impossible to a rational mind, like having the ability to age someone with your mind, suddenly seem possible.

There have been decades of research, like the rubber hand study, on the phenomenon, yet hallucinations continue to intrigue researchers, and there's still no consensus about their basic mechanisms and why they exist.

All we know is that they occur when the brain perceives an outward sensation—vision, sound, or touch—but there is no corresponding external source; it is a failure to distinguish between what is external and what is internal, referred to as self-monitoring theory.

In the same vein, it is precisely because these hallucinations are self-generated that they are so believable and vividly remembered, explained psychology professor Dr. Philip Harvey. It's called the generation effect: "Because those hallucinations were self-generated," Dr. Harvey told me, "you were better able to remember them."

Although people with schizophrenia exhibit cognitive and memory defects, they can remember just as well as healthy people if they are forced to structure the memory themselves. For example, those with schizophrenia best remember lists of words when they are asked to make a story out of the words rather than straightforward and unaided remembering.

Couple this with the fact that these head trips were intensely emotional and would therefore be tagged as important by the hippocampus and amygdala, both of which were affected by my disease. The amygdala, an almond-shaped structure situated atop the hippocampus, located at the sides of the head above the ears in the temporal lobes, is a structure intimately involved in emotion and memory, helping to choose which memories should be kept and which should be discarded, based on which events have traumatized or excited us. The hippocampus tags the memory with context (the hospital room and the purple lady, for example), and the amygdala provides the emotion (fear, excitement, and pain).

When the amygdala stamps the experience with high emotional value, it's more likely to be preserved, a process called encoding, and eventually made into a memory, called consolidation. The hippocampus and amygdala help encode and consolidate the experience, or make it into a memory that can be retrieved later. When any part of this elaborate system is compromised, the memory may not be formed.

Therefore I will likely never forget the time I could age the psychiatrist with my mind, which just shows how fallible memory is. This realization would continue to haunt me.

For instance, I recall with absolute certainty the time I woke up bound by restraints in the hospital's four-person AMU room, watched over by the "purple lady," the scene that opens this book. I vividly remember looking down at my right hand and seeing an orange band that read FLIGHT RISK. My family and friends remembered the same thing, so I took this for granted as a truth. The FLIGHT RISK band to me is a fact.

Yet it turns out it was imaginary. When I spoke to nurses and doctors on my floor, they told me that those bands don't exist. One nurse suggested, "You probably had a FALL RISK band. It wasn't orange; it was yellow." My EEG tapes confirmed this. There is no such thing as an orange FLIGHT RISK band.

"When people think about a past event, they can incorporate new information in their recollection, making a new memory," explained psychologist Elizabeth Loftus. Dr. Loftus has spent a lifetime working on the assumption that memory is often inaccurate. In a 1978 study, now presented in most Psych 101 classes, Dr. Loftus showed participants slides of a red car hitting a pedestrian. Although the photographs established that the car had encountered a stop sign, when Dr. Loftus questioned the subject, she inserted intentionally misleading questions, like, "What color was the *yield* sign?" The study showed that subjects given lead-ing information were more likely to answer incorrectly than those who weren't. These findings have challenged the power of eyewit-ness testimony.

A team of New York–based neuroscientists in 2000 demon-strated this assumption in lab rats by testing to see if memories are constantly altered each time we recall them. The team uncov-ered another step in the memory process, called reconsolidation: when a memory is recalled, it's essentially remade, allowing new (and sometimes wrong) information to filter in. This is normally useful because we need to be able to update our past experiences to reflect present information, but it sometimes creates devious inaccuracies.

Psychology professor Dr. Henry Roedigger calls what hap-pened with the FLIGHT RISK band a form of social contagion: If one person remembers incorrectly and shares this with others, it can spread, like an airborne illness straight out of the movie *Outbreak*.

Did I harbor this false memory? Was I the one who spread it? I am sure I remember vividly seeing the words FLIGHT RISK on my arm. Or am I?

CHAPTER 52
MADAME X

"**O**ur brains make little stories," explained Dr. Chris Morrison, the neuropsychologist who had tested me at the hospital, when I interviewed her in December 2010. "It's possible that when you rehearse things so many times, you start to internalize and believe that you were there. You integrate fragments, scenes of things that you could not truly remember." Like the FLIGHT RISK band.

Similarly, a retrieval mechanism is triggered in the brain when we see something recognizable. Smells or images will instantly transport us back in time, unlocking forgotten memories. A year after I left the hospital, my friend Colleen took me to a nearby pub called Egan's.

The name jarred me. Had I been there before? I couldn't remember.

We walked into the upscale Irish pub and headed toward the bar. Nope. I hadn't been there. But when I stepped into the central dining room area and caught sight of a magnificent low-hanging chandelier, I knew I *had* been here before, right before I got sick, with Stephen, his sister, and her husband before that Ryan Adams show. Not only did I remember being here, but I also remembered what I ordered: fish and chips.

Glistening lard. Piles of gluttonously rich, fat-encrusted french fries. I fought the urge to throw up on the table. I tried to make conversation, but all I could concentrate on was the glistening fish and chips.

I couldn't believe how vividly it came rushing back to me. What else had I forgotten? What else would come back, knock-

246

ing me off balance and reminding me how tenuous my grip on reality was?

Almost every day, something reemerges. It can be something insignificant, like the moss-colored socks at the hospital, or a simple word, like the time in the drugstore when I saw a box of Colace, the stool softener I had taken at the hospital, and the memories of Nurse Adeline came rushing in with it. During these moments, I can't help but think that the other Susannah is calling out to me as if to say, *I may be gone, but I'm not forgotten.* Like the girl in the video: "Please."

But with every memory I recapture, I know there are hundreds, thousands even, that I cannot conjure up. No matter how many doctors I speak with, no matter how many interviews I conduct or how many notebooks I scavenge, there will be many experiences, bits of my life that have vanished.

One morning, a year after I moved in with Stephen, I finally got around to unpacking boxes from my old apartment. I opened a small box filled with an old, broken hair dryer, some curling irons, a few notebooks, and a small brown paper bag. Inside the paper bag was a postcard of a raven-haired woman. It was a famous painting, and I knew I had seen it before, but it held no context for me:

The woman stands majestically in profile, which exaggerates her downward-sloping nose and long forehead. Her pale skin contrasts sharply against the blackness of her evening dress, which leaves her shoulders bare, only two jeweled straps holding the dress in place. She supports her unnatural pose by leaning the weight of her body on the tips of her right fingers, which are propped against a wooden table; her other hand lifts the hem of her skirt in a queenly fashion. It's a seductive and artificial pose. To me, she looks at once both haughty and sick, as if too arrogant to admit that she is deathly ill.

There was something oddly magnetic about this woman, so different from the entirely alien push-and-pull mixture of attraction and repulsion that I felt with Dr. Bailey's distorted version of a human form, that *Carota* picture. Taking in this woman, an ancient feeling surged through me, a prickly, exhilarating sensation that I could trace to my childhood. After a moment, I found the source: I had the same feeling when I used to snoop through my mom's closet when I was a child. I stared at the picture for several more minutes, trying to understand the link between the picture and that forgotten memory, before I could pry myself away long enough to turn the postcard over.

It was John Singer Sargent's *Madame X,* from 1884. Also in the bag was a receipt for the date of purchase. I had bought the $1.63 postcard at the Metropolitan Museum of Art on February 17, 2009, shortly before my first breakdown at work. There was not one shred, one iota, one *shard* of memory that connected me with that museum visit. I could not recall going to the Met that February day. I could not remember standing in front of the painting or what had originally engrossed me about this powerful yet vulnerable woman.

Or maybe on some level, I can remember. I like to believe what Friedrich Nietzsche said: "The existence of forgetting has never been proved: we only know that some things do not come to our mind when we want them to."

Maybe it's not gone but is somewhere in the recesses of my mind, waiting for the proper cues to be called back up. So far that hasn't happened, which just makes me wonder: What else have I lost along the way? And is it actually lost or just hidden?

Some buried feeling unites me fiercely with that painting. I have since mounted it on the wall above me in the room where I write, and often I find myself staring off at it when I'm lost in thought. Maybe, even though "I" was not there to experience it for the first time, some part of me nevertheless was present during that museum visit, and maybe for that entire lost month. That idea comforts me.

CHAPTER 53

THE PURPLE LADY

Nearly two years after my release from the epilepsy floor at New York University Langone Medical Center, I return for a visit.

I walk up First Avenue toward the purple NYU sign that hangs on the massive gray hospital building in the distance. I press against the sluggish revolving door, made to move slowly to accommodate those in wheelchairs, which opens up into the hospital's modern lobby. Doctors in white lab coats walk briskly past patients and various drug salesmen who look like aged frat boys. Somber visitors holding plastic "Patient's Belongings" bags disappear into the background. Automatic Purell hand sanitizer dispensers dot the entranceways. I walk past the admitting station where I had my seizure, though all I can remember from that day is the hot cappuccino I'd bought moments before I was admitted.

I get on an elevator that takes me to the twelfth floor. My thoughts wander to my parents and Stephen, who took this very trip several times a day for a month. Incredible.

Strangely, though, everything looks unfamiliar. None of the nurses recognize me. I walk through the corridor and past the nurses' station. No one looks up. A man sprawled out on the hallway floor is making a gurgling sound. The nurses behind the station run past me toward him. I follow behind them. The older man thrashes, emitting primitive guttural grunts. A team of nurses holds him down as a security guard lifts him onto a gurney. The man's gown is open below his belly button. I turn away from the sight. A nurse in green scrubs walks by me.

"Is this the epilepsy unit?" I ask her.

"No. You've got the wrong floor. This is the east wing. Epilepsy is on the west wing, same floor." Well, at least this time it wasn't my memory playing tricks on me.

I return to the lobby and take another elevator up, but again find, to my disappointment, that nothing looks familiar. Then the smell hits me: a combination of alcohol-soaked cotton swabs with a sweet muskiness. This is the place; it has to be. Then I see her. The purple lady. She stares at me. But this time it's not with horror or pity or fear. In her eyes I'm a normal, healthy person, just someone whose face she is struggling to place.

I smile. "Do you remember me?" I ask.

"I'm not sure," she admits. There's that same Jamaican accent. "What's your name?"

"Susannah Cahalan."

Her eyes widen. "Oh, yes, I remember you. I do remember you." She smiles. "I'm sure it's you, but you look so different. You look all better."

Before I know it, we're embracing. The scent of her body is like Purell. Images flood through my mind's eye: my father feeding me oatmeal, my mom wringing her hands and looking nervously out of the window, Stephen arriving with that leather briefcase. I should be crying, but I smile instead.

The purple lady kisses me softly on the cheek.

Afterword

I returned to NYU a year later. This was not another book-related exhumation, but to visit a patient of Dr. Najjar's who had recently been diagnosed with the same disease that struck me. When I reached room 1203, just down the floor from where I had lived for that month, I recognized the patient's parents by the hungry, exhausted look in their eyes. They led me into the room and I saw her—me—lying prone in the bed.

I saw a storminess in her heavily lidded eyes, but a deadness also that jolted me into the past. *This is what I looked like.* She gripped the side rails, excited, confused, yearning to touch me, the recovered one. But her body wouldn't comply; it was too rigid and uncertain. But she could move enough to hug me. Her skin radiated heat; I could feel each of her ribs.

She looked past me, repeating, "I can't believe you're here," as if to say, I can't believe you're real.

Her parents later explained the circumstances that landed their daughter in Dr. Najjar's care. It was thanks to Dr. Bailey, the same doctor who had believed I was suffering from alcohol withdrawal. They consulted him after she had been admitted to a psychiatric ward. He suggested they reach out to Dr. Najjar about a disease he had read in the pages of *Neurology.* He did not admit that he had missed my case, but he had obviously learned from it.

What used to be called a "zebra" (in doctor parlance, a very rare disease) is now increasingly recognized and swiftly treated. When I was diagnosed, it was believed that 90 percent of cases went undiagnosed. Now many doctors know to test for it, and if it is found early and treated aggressively, 81 percent of patients recover fully, a staggeringly high figure considering how utterly devastating the disease appears at its height. The girl I visited at NYU, for example, is back to work, living on her own, and as vibrant as ever.

Despite all the progress since I was diagnosed in 2009, there's much more to be done. The mortality rate is still at about 7 percent. And some do not recover fully. What triggers the disease (in those without teratomas) remains unknown. New variants are being discovered; as of this writing, there are seven types.

I've made it my mission to share my story with as many people as possible. I've visited universities, hospitals, and psychiatric institutions presenting my case. I've also helped to start a new nonprofit foundation called the Autoimmune Encephalitis Alliance, devoted to research and spreading awareness, with the ultimate goal that everyone receive the same quality of care that I did. You can learn more at www.aealliance.org.

I believe this book has lent many people legitimacy to their suffering. I've given them a name for what ails them, and for others who still don't have a name, I've given them hope.

Someone once asked, "If you could take it all back, would you?"

At the time I didn't know. Now I do. I wouldn't take that terrible experience back for anything in the world. Too much light has come out of my darkness.

NOTES

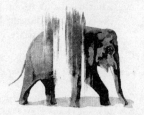

CHAPTER 1: BEDBUG BLUES

8 those suffering from parasitosis: Nancy C. Hinkle, "Delusory Parasitosis," *American Entomologist* 46, no. 1 (2000): 17–25, http://www.ent.uga.edu/pubs/delusory.pdf (accessed August 2, 2011).

9 releasing millions of virus particles: Vincent Racaniello, "Virology 101," *Virology Blog: About Viruses and Diseases,* http://www.virology.ws/virology-101/ (accessed March 1, 2011). Robert Kulwich, "Flu Attack! How the Virus Invades Your Body," *NPR.org* [blog], October 23, 2009 (accessed March 1, 2011).

CHAPTER 4: THE WRESTLER

21 "I used to try to forget about you": Robert D. Siegel, *The Wrestler,* directed by Darren Aronofsky, Fox Searchlight, 2008.

CHAPTER 7: ON THE ROAD AGAIN

39 "That's nice to have at seven in the morning": "Basking in Basque Country," *Spain . . . on the Road Again,* PBS, New York, original broadcast date October 18, 2008.

CHAPTER 8: OUT-OF-BODY EXPERIENCE

42 complex partial seizures: Epilepsy Foundation, "Temporal Lobe Epilepsy," Epilepsyfoundation.org, http://www.epilepsyfoundation.org/aboutepilepsy/syndromes/temporallobeepilepsy.cfm (accessed March 1, 2011). Temkin Owsei, *The Falling Sickness: A History of Epilepsy from the Greeks to the Beginnings of Modern Neurology* (Baltimore: Johns Hopkins University Press, 1971).

42 range from a "Christmas morning": Alice W. Flaherty, *The Midnight Disease: The Drive to Write, Writer's Block and the Creative Brain* (New York: Houghton Mifflin, 2004), 27.

42 religious experiences: Akira Ogata and Taihei Miyakawa, "Religious Experience in Epileptic Patients with Focus on Ictal-Related Episodes," *Psychiatry and Clinical Neurosciences* 52 (1998): 321–325, http://onlinelibrary.wiley.com/doi/10.1046/j.1440-1819.1998.00397.x/pdf.

42 A small subset of those with temporal lobe epilepsy: Shahar Arzy, Gregor Thut, Christine Mohr, Christoph M. Michel, and Olaf Blanke, "Neural Basis of Embodiment: Distinct Contributions of Temporoparietal Junction and Extrastriate Body Area," *Journal of Neuroscience* 26 (2006): 8074–8081.

CHAPTER 9: A TOUCH OF MADNESS

47 best places to live in America by *Money* magazine: CNN Money, "Best Places to Live: 2005," Money.CNN.com, http://money.cnn.com/magazines/moneymag/bplive/2005/snapshots/30683.html (accessed Thursday, April 12, 2012).

48 "a brain disorder that causes unusual shifts in moods": National Institutes of Health, "Bipolar Disorder," NIH.gov, http://www.nimh.nih.gov/health/publications/bipolar-disorder/nimh-bipolar-adults.pdf (accessed March 14, 2009).

48 Jim Carrey, Winston Churchill, Mark Twain, Vivien Leigh, Ludwig van Beethoven, Tim Burton: *Bipolar Disorder Today,* "Famous People with Bipolar Disorder," Mental-Health-Today.com, http://www.mental-health-today.com/bp/famous_people.htm (accessed March 14, 2009).

CHAPTER 15: THE CAPGRAS DELUSION

77 her husband had become a "double": Orin Devinsky, "Delusional Misidentifications and Duplications," *Neurology* 72 (2009): 80–87.

77 revealed that Capgras delusions: Jad Abumrad and Robert Krulwich, "Seeing Imposters: When Loved Ones Suddenly Aren't," NPR, March 30, 2010, http://www.npr.org/templates/story/story.php?storyId=124745692 (accessed May 4, 2011). V. S. Ramachandran and Sandra Blakeslee, *Phantoms in the Brain: Probing the Mysteries of the Human Mind* (New York: Morrow, 1998), 161–171.

CHAPTER 16: POSTICTAL FURY

81 twelve hours or as long as three months: Orin Devinsky, "Postictal Psychosis: Common, Dangerous, and Treatable," *Epilepsy Currents,* February 26, 2008, 31–34. Kenneth Alper et al., "Premorbid Psychiatric Risk Factors for Postictal Psychosis," *Journal of Neuropsychiatry and Clinical Neuroscience* 13 (2001): 492–499. Akira Ogata and Taihei Miyakawa, "Religious Experience in Epileptic Patients with Focus on Ictal-Related Episodes," *Psychiatry and Clinical Neuroscience* 52 (1998): 321–325.

81 "postictal fury": S. J. Logsdail and B. K. Toone, "Post-Ictal Psychoses: A Clinical and Phenomenological Description," *British Journal of Psychiatry* 152 (1988): 246–252.

81 A quarter of psychotic people: Michael Trimble, Andy Kanner, and Bettina Schmitz, "Postictal Psychosis," *Epilepsy and Behavior* 19 (2010): 159–161.

CHAPTER 17: MULTIPLE PERSONALITY DISORDER

83 I was within the age range for psychotic breaks: The New York Times Health Guide, "Schizophrenia," *Health.nytimes.com,* http://health.nytimes.com/health/guides/disease/schizophrenia/risk-factors.html (accessed February 20, 2010).

83 dissociative identity disorder (DID): "Dissociative Identity Disorder," in American Psychiatric Association, *Diagnostic and Statistical Manual of Mental Disorders—IV (Text Revision)* (Washington, D.C.: American Psychiatric Association, 2 000), 526–529.

85 On of a scale from 1 (most dire cases) to 100: "Bipolar Disorder," in ibid.

CHAPTER 18: BREAKING NEWS

86 "Like a bolt from the blue": P. A. Pichot, "A Comparison of Different National Concepts of Schizoaffective Psychosis," in *Schizoaffective Psychoses* (Berlin: Springer-Verlag, 1986), 8–16. A. Marneros and M. T. Tsuang, "Schizoaffective Questions and Directions," in *Schizoaffective Psychoses* (Berlin: Springer-Verlag, 1986).

87 "uninterrupted period of illness during": American Psychiatric Association, *Diagnostic and Statistical Manual of Mental Disorders—IV (Text Revision)* (Washington, D.C.: American Psychiatric Association, 2000), 319–323.

CHAPTER 21: DEATH WITH INTERRUPTIONS

102 In 1933, a bicycle struck seven-year-old Henry Gustav Molaison: Luke Dittrich, "The Brain That Changed Everything," Esquire.com, October 5, 2010, www.esquire.com/features/henry-molaison-brain-1110 (accessed May 8, 2011). "Histopathological Examination of the Brain of Amnesiac Patient H.M.," *Brain Observatory,* August 18, 2010, http://thebrainobservatory.ucsd.edu/content/histopathological-examination-brain-amnesic-patient-hm (accessed May 8, 2011). William Beecher Scoville and Brenda Milner, "Loss of Recent Memory after Bilateral Hippocampal Lesions," *Journal of Neurology, Neurosurgery and Psychiatry* 20 (1957): 11–21. Benedict Carey, "H.M., an Unforgettable Amnesiac, Dies at 82," *New York Times,* December 5, 2008, http://www.nytimes.com/2008/12/05/us/05hm.html?pagewanted=all (accessed May 8, 2011).

102 "Clive was under the constant impression": Deborah Wearing, *Forever Today: A True Story of Lost Memory and Never-Ending Love* (London: Corgi, 2006).

103 "I haven't heard anything": Oliver Sacks, "The Abyss: Music and Amnesia," *New Yorker,* September 24, 2007, http://www.newyorker.com/reporting/2007/09/24/070924fa_fact_sacks (accessed September 13, 2011).

CHAPTER 22: A BEAUTIFUL MESS

107 At the top of the spinal cord and at the underside of the brain: Michael O'Shea, *The Brain: A Very Short Introduction* (Oxford: Oxford University Press, 2005). Rita Carter, Susan Aldridge, Martyn Page, and Steve Parker, *The Human Brain Book* (London: DK Adult, 2009). Stephen G. Waxman, *Clinical Neuroanatomy, Twenty-Sixth Edition* (New York: McGraw Hill, 2010).

107 "The brain is a monstrous, beautiful mess": William F. Allman, *Apprentices of Wonder: Inside the Neural Network Revolution* (New York: Bantam, 1989), 3.

CHAPTER 24: IVIG

116 IVIG is made up of serum antibodies: Falk Nimmerjahn and Jeffrey V. Ravetch, "The Anti-Inflammatory Activity of IgG: The Intravenous IgG Paradox," *Journal of Experimental Medicine* 204 (2007): 11–15. Arturo Casadevall, Ekaterina Dadachova, and Liise-Anne Pirofski, "Passive Antibody Therapy for Infectious Diseases," *Nature Reviews Microbiology* 2 (2004): 695–703. Noah S. Scheinfeld, "Intravenous Immunoglobulin," *Medscape Reference,* http://emedicine.medscape.com/article/210367-overview (accessed May 8, 2011).

116 Antibodies are created by the body's immune system: John M. Dwyer, *The Body at War: The Story of Our Immune System* (Sydney, Australia: Allen & Unwin, 1994), 28–52. S. Jane Flint, Lynn W. Enquist, Vincent R. Racaniello, and A. M. Skalka, *Principles of Virology: Molecular Biology, Pathogenesis, and Control of Animal Viruses, Third Edition* (Washington, D.C.: American Society of Microbiology, 2009), 86–130. Noel R. Rose and Ian R. Mackay, eds., *The Autoimmune Diseases, Fourth Edition* (St. Louis, Mo.: Elsevier, 2006). Lauren Sompayrac, *How the Immune System Works, Third Edition* (Oxford: Blackwell, 2008). Massoud Mahmoudi, *Immunology Made Ridiculously Simple* (Miami: Med Master, 2009). Robert G. Lahita, *Women and Autoimmune Disease: The Mysterious Ways Your Body Betrays Itself* (New York: Morrow, 2004).

116 ten days versus the innate system's minutes or hours: Vincent Racaniello, "Innate Immune Defenses," Virology.ws, http://www.virology.ws/2009/06/03/innate-immune-defenses (accessed March 11, 2010). Vincent Racaniello, "Adaptive Immune Defenses," Virology.ws, http://www.virology.ws/2009/07/03/adaptive-immune-defenses (accessed March 11, 2010).

116 collateral damage of these internal battles: Lauren Sompayrac, *How the Immune System Works, Third Edition* (Oxford: Blackwell, 2008). Massoud Mahmoudi, *Immunology Made Ridiculously Simple* (Miami: Med Master, 2009). Robert G. Lahita, *Women and Autoimmune Disease: The Mysterious Ways Your Body Betrays Itself* (New York: Morrow, 2004).

117 plasma cells that create antibodies: John M. Dwyer, *The Body at War: The Story of Our Immune System* (Sydney, Australia: Allen & Unwin,

1994), 28–52. S. Jane Flint, Lynn W. Enquist, Vincent R. Racaniello, and A. M. Skalka, *Principles of Virology: Molecular Biology, Pathogenesis, and Control of Animal Viruses, Third Edition* (Washington, D.C.: American Society of Microbiology, 2009), 86–130. Noel R. Rose and Ian R. Mackay, eds., *The Autoimmune Diseases: Fourth Edition* (St. Louis: Elsevier, 2006). Lauren Sompayrac, *How the Immune System Works, Third Edition* (Oxford: Blackwell, 2008). Massoud Mahmoudi, *Immunology Made Ridiculously Simple* (Miami: Med Master, 2009). Robert G. Lahita, *Women and Autoimmune Disease: The Mysterious Ways Your Body Betrays Itself* (New York: Morrow, 2004).

119 WIRED 'N MIRED: Brendan T. Carroll, Christopher Thomas, Kameshwari Jayanti, John M. Hawkins, and Carrie Burbage, "Treating Persistent Catatonia When Benzodiazepines Fail," *Current Psychiatry* 4 (2005): 59.

CHAPTER 26: THE CLOCK

130 Although developed in the mid-1950s: Janus Kremer, "Clock Drawing in Dementia: A Critical Review," *Revista Neurologica Argentina* 27 (2002): 223–227.

132 The healthy brain enables vision: Francesco Pavani, Elisabetta Ladavas, and Jon Driver, "Auditory and Multisensory Aspects of Visuospatial Neglect," *Trends in Cognitive Sciences* 7 (2008): 407–414. V. S. Ramachandran and Sandra Blakeslee, *Phantoms in the Brain: Probing the Mysteries of the Human Mind* (New York: Morrow, 1998), 115–125. V. S. Ramachandran, *The Tell-Tale Brain: A Neuroscientist's Quest for What Makes Us Human* (New York: Norton, 2011), 1–21. Michael O'Shea, *The Brain: A Very Short Introduction* (Oxford: Oxford University Press, 2005). Rita Carter, Susan Aldridge, Martyn Page, and Steve Parker, *The Human Brain Book* (London: DK Adult, 2009). Stephen G. Waxman, *Clinical Neuroanatomy, Twenty-Sixth Edition* (New York: McGraw-Hill, 2010).

133 visual indifference: V. S. Ramachandran and Sandra Blakeslee, *Phantoms in the Brain: Probing the Mysteries of the Human Mind* (New York: Morrow, 1998), 118.

CHAPTER 28: SHADOWBOXER

143 The blood-brain barrier (BBB): Davis Lab, "History of the Blood Brain Barrier," University of Arizona, http://davislab.med.arizona.edu/content/history-blood-brain-barrier (accessed April 23, 2011).

144 These steroids, called corticosteroids: Julia C. Buckingham, "Glucocorticoids: Exemplars of Multi-Tasking," *British Journal of Pharmacology* 147 (2006): S258—S268. Mayo Clinic Staff, "Prednisone and Other Corticosteroids: Balance the Risks and Benefits," MayoClinic.com, http://www.mayoclinic.com/health/steriods/HQ01431 (accessed May 8, 2011). Peter J. Barnes, "How Corticosteroids Control Inflammation: Quintiles Prize Lecture 2005," *British Journal of Pharmacology* 148 (2006): 245–254.

CHAPTER 29: DALMAU'S DISEASE

146 paraneoplastic syndrome: National Institute of Neurological Disorders and Stroke, "NINDS Paraneoplastic Syndrome Information Page," National Institutes of Health, http://www.ninds.nih.gov/disorders/paraneoplastic/paraneoplastic.htm (accessed March 2, 2011). Roberta Vitaliani, Warren Mason, Beau Ances, Theodore Zwerdling, Zhilong Jiang, and Josep Dalmau, "Paraneoplastic Encephalitis, Psychiatric Symptoms, and Hypoventilation in Ovarian Teratomas," *Annals of Neurology* 58 (2005): 594–604.

149 NMDA (N-methyl-D-aspartate acid) receptors are vital to learning: David J. Linden, *The Accidental Mind: How Brain Evolution Has Given Us Love, Memory, Dreams and God* (Cambridge, Mass.: Belknap Press of Harvard University Press, 2007), 107–144. Fei Li and Joe Z. Tsien, "Memory and NMDA Receptors," *New England Journal of Medicine* 361 (2009): 302–303.

150 "knockout mice" without NMDA receptors: Wade Roush, "New Knockout Mice Point to Molecular Basis of Memory," *Science* 275 (1997), www.bio.davidson.edu/courses/molbio/restricted/knockbrain/BrainKO.html (accessed May 18, 2011). Zhenzhong Cui, Huimin Wang, Yuansheng Tan, Kimberly A. Zaia, Shuqin Zhang, and Joe Z. Tsein, "Inducible and Reversible NR1 Knockout Reveals Crucial Role of the NMDA Receptor in Preserving Remote Memories in the Brain," *Neuron* 41 (2004): 781–793. Laure Rondi-Reig, Megan Libbey, Howard Eichenbaum, and Susumu Tonegawa, "CA1-Specific NMDA Receptor Knockout Mice Are Deficient in Solving Nonspatial Transverse Patterning Task," *Proceedings of the National Academy of Sciences* 98 (2001): 3543–3548.

150 This second article identified twelve women: Josep Dalmau et al., "Paraneoplastic Anti-N-Methyl-D-Aspartate Receptor Encephalitis Associated with Ovarian Teratoma," *Annals of Neurology* 61 (2007): 25–36.

CHAPTER 31: THE BIG REVEAL

157 For 70 percent of patients, the disorder begins innocuously, with normal flulike symptoms: Josep Dalmau et al., "Clinical Experience and Laboratory Investigations in Patients with Anti-NMDAR Encephalitis," *Lancet Neurology* 10 (2011): 63–74.

159 75 percent of patients recover fully or maintain only mild side effects: Josep Dalmau et al., "Clinical Experience and Laboratory Investigations in Patients with Anti-NMDAR Encephalitis," *Lancet Neurology* 10 (2011): 63–74.

158 late 1800s, a German doctor christened it "teratoma": Elizabeth Svoboda, "Monster Tumors Show Scientific Potential in War against Cancer," *New York Times,* June 6, 2006, http://www.nytimes.com/2006/06/06/health/06tera.html (accessed May 1, 2011).

CHAPTER 33: HOMECOMING

167 stages of recovery often occur in reverse order: Josep Dalmau et al., "Clinical Experience and Laboratory Investigations in Patients with Anti-NMDAR Encephalitis," *Lancet Neurology* 10 (2011): 63–74.

CHAPTER 34: CALIFORNIA DREAMIN'

170 Swedish dairy cream separator created in the late 1800s: T. J. Hamblin, "Apheresis Therapy: Spin-Drying the Blood," *British Medical Journal* 285 (1982): 1136–1137. Dianne M. Cearlock and David Gerteisen, "Therapeutic Plasmapheresis for Autoimmune Diseases: Advances and Outcomes," *Medical Laboratory Observer,* November 2010, http://www.mlo-online.com/articles/nov00.pdf (accessed May 2011).

CHAPTER 39: WITHIN NORMAL LIMITS

193 Often those with neurological issues cannot readily identify: Rhawn Joseph, *Neuropsychiatry, Neuropsychology, Clinical Neuroscience* (Orlando, Fla.: Academic Press, 2000), http://brainmind.com/Agnosia.html.

CHAPTER 40: UMBRELLA

195 frontal lobes are largely responsible for complex executive functions: Michael O'Shea, *The Brain: A Very Short Introduction* (Oxford: Oxford University Press, 2005). Rita Carter, Susan Aldridge, Martyn Page, and Steve Parker, *The Human Brain Book* (London: DK Adult, 2009).

195 "ice pick" lobotomy: "My Lobotomy: Henry Dully's Journey," *All Things Considered,* NPR.org, November 16, 2005, http://www.npr.org/templates/story/story.php?storyId=5014080 (accessed May 13, 2011). Shanna Freeman, "How Lobotomies Work," HowStuffWorks.com, http://science.howstuffworks.com/environmental/life/human-biology/lobotomy3.htm (accessed May 13, 2011).

CHAPTER 43: NDMA

207 *New York Times Magazine* "Diagnosis" column: Lisa Sanders, "Diagnosis: Brain Drain," *New York Times Magazine,* November 9, 2008, http://query.nytimes.com/gst/fullpage.html?res=9C05E7DA1F3BF93AA35752C1A96E9C8B63.

CHAPTER 47: THE EXORCIST

221 Dr. Guillaume Sébire noticed an unusual pattern: Guillaume Sébire et al., "Coma Associated with Intense Bursts of Abnormal Movements and Long-Lasting Cognitive Disturbances: An Acute Encephalopathy of Obscure Origin," *Journal of Pediatrics* 121 (1992): 845–851.

221 1981 by Robert Delong and colleagues, described: Robert G. Delong et al., "Acquired Reversible Autistic Syndrome in Acute Encephalopathic Illness in Children," *Child Neurology* 38 (1981): 191–194.

222 40 percent of patients diagnosed with this disease are children: Josep Dalmau et al., "Clinical Experience and Laboratory Investigations in Patients with Anti-NMDAR Encephalitis," *Lancet Neurology* 10 (2011): 63–74.

222 thirteen-year-old girl from Tennessee displayed: Emily Bregel, "Chattanooga: Teen Has 'Miraculous' Recovery from an Unusual Tumor Disorder," TimesFreePress.com, June 11, 2009, http://timesfreepress.com/news/2009/jun/11/chattanooga-teen-has-miraculous-recovery-unusual-t/?local.

223 what is known as echolalia: Guillaume Sébire, "In Search of Lost Time: From Demonic Possession to Anti-NMDAR Encephalitis," *Annals of Neurology* 66 (2009): 11–8. Nicole R. Florance and Josep Dalmau, "Reply to: In Search of Lost Time: From 'Demonic Possession to Anti-NMDAR Encephalitis,'" *Annals of Neurology* 67 (2010): 142–143.

225 a nineteen-year-old woman: Souhel Najjar, D. Pearlman, D. Zagzag, J. Golfinos, and O. Devinsky, "Glutamic Acid Decarboxylase Autoantibody Syndrome Presenting as Schizophrenia," *Neurologist* 18 (2012): 88–91.

226 the rate of misdiagnoses: David Leonhardt, "Why Doctors So Often Get It Wrong," *New York Times,* February 22, 2006, http://www.nytimes.com/2006/02/22/business/22leonhardt.html.

CHAPTER 48: SURVIVOR'S GUILT

229 one hundred different kinds of autoimmune diseases: American Autoimmune Related Diseases Association and National Coalition of Autoimmune Patient Groups, "The Cost Burden of Autoimmune Disease: The Latest Front in the War on Healthcare Spending" (Eastpointe, Mich.: American Autoimmune Related Diseases Association, 2011). Autoimmune Diseases Coordinating Committee, "Autoimmune Diseases Research" (Bethesda, Md.: National Institutes of Health, March 2005).

231 20 to 30 percent of survivors develop it: Gwen Adshead, "Psychological Therapies for Post-Traumatic Stress Disorder," *British Journal of Psychiatry* 177 (2000): 144–148.

CHAPTER 50: ECSTATIC

240 relapses happen in about 20 percent of cases: Josep Dalmau et al., "Clinical Experience and Laboratory Investigations in Patients with Anti-NMDAR Encephalitis," *Lancet Neurology* 10 (2011): 63–74.

CHAPTER 51: FLIGHT RISK?

242 In 2010, a Cambridge University study: Hannah L. Morgan, Danielle C. Turner, Philip R. Corlett, Anthony R. Absalom, Ram Adapa, Fernando S. Arana, Jennifer Pigott, Jenny Gardner, Jessica Everitt, Patrick Haggard,

and Paul C. Fletcher, "Exploring the Impact of Ketamine on the Experience of Illusory Body Ownership," *Biological Psychiatry* 69, no. 1 (2011): 35–41.

243 self-monitoring theory: Sharon Begley, "The Schizophrenic Mind," *Newsweek*, March 11, 2002, www.newsweek.com/2002/03/10/the-schizophrenic-mind.print.html (accessed April 21, 2011). Dominic H. Ffytche, "The Hodology of a Hallucinations," *Cortex* 44 (2008): 1067–1083.

243 generation effect: Philip D. Harvey et al., "Cortical and Subcortical Cognitive Deficits in Schizophrenia: Convergence of Classifications Based on Language and Memory Skill Areas," *Journal of Clinical and Experimental Neuropsychology* 24 (2002): 55–66. Carol A. Tamminga, Ana D. Stan, and Anthony D. Wagner, "The Hippocampal Formation in Schizophrenia," *American Journal of Psychiatry* 167 (2010): 1178–1193. Daphna Shohamy, Perry Mihalakos, Ronald Chin, Binu Thomas, Anthony D. Wagner, and Carol Tamminga, "Learning and Generalization in Schizophrenia: Effects of Disease and Antipsychotic Drug Treatment," *Biological Psychiatry* 67 (2010): 926–932.

243 amygdala, an almond-shaped structure situated atop the hippocampus: Michael O'Shea, *The Brain: A Very Short Introduction* (Oxford: Oxford University Press, 2005). Rita Carter, Susan Aldridge, Martyn Page, and Steve Parker, *The Human Brain Book* (London: DK Adult, 2009). Elizabeth A. Phelps and Tali Sharot, "How (and Why) Emotion Enhances Subjective Sense of Recollection," *Current Directions in Psychological Sciences* 17 (2008): 147–152, http://www.psych.nyu.edu/phelpslab/papers/08_CDPS_V17No2_147.pdf. Joseph E. LeDoux, "Emotion Circuits in the Brain," *Annual Reviews of Neuroscience* 23 (2000): 155–185.

244 help encode and consolidate: Jesse Rissman and Anthony D. Wagner, "Distributed Representations in Memory: Insights from Functional Brain Imaging," *Annual Review of Psychology* 63 (2012): 101–128. Richard C. Mohs, "How Human Memory Works," HowStuffWorks.com, http://science.howstuffworks.com/environmental/life/human-biology/human-memory.htm.

244 Dr. Loftus has spent a lifetime: William Saletan, "The Memory Doctor: The Future of False Memories," Slate.com, June 4, 2010, http://www.slate.com/articles/health_and_science/the_memory_doctor/2010/06/the_memory_doctor.single.html.

245 A team of New York–based neuroscientists in 2000 demonstrated this assumption in lab rats: Greg Miller, "How Our Brains Make Memories," *Smithsonian*, May 2010, http://www.smithsonianmag.com/science-nature/How-Our-Brains-Make-Memories.html. "Big Think Interview with Joseph LeDoux," BigThink.com, June 9, 2010, http://bigthink.com/josephledoux.

ACKNOWLEDGMENTS

Of course, it's been said before: I could never have done this without all of you. But I believe that, in my case, this cliché rings true. I can say, in all honesty, that without the incredible people who make up my life, I would not be here right now writing these words.

I am forever grateful for the love and support provided to me by the fighters, my family: my mother, my father, Stephen, and James. Thank you also to my extended family: Allen Goldman, Giselle Cahalan, Hannah Green, Len Green, and Ana Coelho, who never lost sight of me, even during my darkest hours. And to Stephen's "Good Turkey" kin and his parents John Grywalski and Jane O'Malley for raising such a remarkable son. You all are my rocks. I continue to thrive because of you.

How do I thank my brilliant and selfless Drs. House: Dr. Souhel Najjar and Dr. Josep Dalmau? I'll keep it simple: thank you for saving my life. And, if that wasn't enough, thank you both for contributing so much of your precious time to this project, for explaining the vagaries of our brains and immune systems, and for vetting the manuscript. Thank you also to the New York University Langone Medical Center, specifically Dr. Sabrina Khan, Dr. Jung Hwan Ahn, Dr. Jeffery Friedman, Dr. Werner Doyle, Karen Gendal, Tamara Ricaforte, Laura Dumbrava, Dr. Hilary Bertisch, nurse Steve Schoenberg, Dr. Orrin Devinsky, Dorie Klissas, and Craig Andrews. As my parents said in their note: "I cannot think of more meaningful work than what you do every day."

Then there's the whole lonely and terrifying business of sitting down and writing a book. I am so fortunate to have the super-agent duo of Larry Weissman and Sascha Alper representing me. They believed in me from moment one, and continued to guide me through the difficult process of writing. Along the way you both have come to mean more to me than mere business associate: you're family.

Thank you to Free Press, a publishing house that has become a home to me over the past two years. To the immensely gifted Hilary Redmon, who selected and edited my manuscript: thank you for seeing that special something in my story, loving the science as much as I do, and kneading the story into a narrative. Then there's the exceptional Millicent Bennett, who through her deft editorial flourishes and probing questions took the book to the next level, making it sing in ways I could never have dreamed. Thank you also to publicists Jill Siegel and Carisa Hays for their belief in the importance of my story and to Chloe Perkins, who put in a lot of late nights making this a better book. Thank you to the whole Free Press team: Suzanne Donahue, Nicole Judge, Paul O'Halloran, Edith Lewis, Beverly Miller, Claire Kelley, Alanna Ramirez, Sydney Tanigawa, Laura Tatham, Kevin McCahill, Brittany Dulac, Kelly Roberts, and Erin Reback. And, finally, to Dominick Anfuso and Martha Levin for putting such faith in me and creating such an amazingly supportive place for writers.

To my dazzling illustrator Morgan Schweitzer: you got it instantly, and your illustrations breathe such life into my work. My appreciation to the virtuosic Meehan Crist, who not only helped me get a grasp on the complexities, but also guided me toward finding my voice.

Thank you to the patient and helpful experts: Dr. Rita Balice-Gordon at the University of Pennsylvania, who has a special knack for explaining abstractions; Dr. Chris Morrison at the New York University Medical Center, who was so crucial to my understanding of the brain's "glitches"; Dr. Vincent Racaniello at Columbia University, who shared his knowledge of the awesomeness of viruses; Dr. Philip Harvey at the University of Miami, who showed me how my disease fits within the study of schizophrenia;

Dr. Robert Lahita at Newark Beth Israel, who spent hours on the phone bantering about phagocytes; Dr. David Linden at Johns Hopkins University, who patiently explained to me the role of NMDA receptors in the brain; Dr. Joel Pachter at the University of Connecticut, who revealed how the blood-brain barrier works; and, finally, Dr. Henry Roediger III at Washington University in St. Louis and Dr. Elizabeth Loftus at the University of Washington, for explaining false-memory research.

I am grateful to the librarians of the library at the New York Academy of Medicine and at the New York Public Library, and to my fellow science writers at Columbia's NeuWrite group who helped me accurately navigate through the more intricate scientific passages.

To the incredibly brave survivors and families who have so generously made me a part of their lives: Nesrin Shaheen and her daughter Sonia Gramcko; Emily, Bill, and Grace Gavigan; Sandra Reali; Cheryl, Tony, and Jayden Liuzza; Kiera Givens Echols; Angie McGowan; Donna Harris Zulauf; Annalisa Meier and her parents; and so many others.

To Paul McPolin, my straight-shooting *Post* editor, you are, as I said, a brilliant editor, and your work and generosity show in these pages. To my *Post* neighbor Maureen Callahan, who spent many nights listening to me babble over martinis: your insights show on these pages as well. And to Angela Montefinise, who told me the book was "great" when it was far from it, who brought me a cheeseburger in the hospital, who rescued my blue-haired stray, Dusty: I am forever in your debt. And thank you to the extraordinary Julie Stapen not only for bringing some needed levity (with her now infamous "poop" picture) but also for spending two hours patiently shooting me in search of the perfect author photo.

Thank you to Katie Strauss for the stuffed rat, Jennifer Arms for the pumpernickel bagel, Lindsey Derrington for visiting me all the way from St. Louis, Colleen Gutwein for those gorgeous pictures of Cambodia, Mackenzie Dawson for her Sartre quote, and Ginger Adams Otis and Zach Haberman for taking care of Dusty when I wasn't able to.

To the *New York Post,* and especially the Sunday staff, which has been so supportive during my illness and throughout the writing of this book. The *Post*'s cast of characters are among my closest friends. Thank you to the following who have helped in one way or another with the writing of this book: Jim Fanelli, Hasani Gittens, Sue Edelman, Liz Pressman, Isabel Vincent, Rob Walsh, and Kirsten Fleming. Thanks to Steve Lynch, who edited the article "My Mysterious Lost Month of Madness," on which this book is based, and to my first editor, Lauren Ramsby, who taught me the value of asking that extra "why."

To the friends and family who offered up their valued perspectives: the Goldmans, the Fasanos, Rosemarie Terenzio, Bryan Cirelli, Jay Turon, Sarah Nurre, Frank Fenimore, Kelsey Kiefer, Calle Gartside, David Bernard, Kristy Schwarzman, Beth Starker, and Jeff Vines. And thank you to Preston Browning, who offered me a place to write at his charming Wellspring House, which has become my second home.

And, finally, thank you to the "purple lady," whose name I still don't know.

ILLUSTRATION CREDITS

ABOUT THE AUTHOR

Susannah Cahalan began her investigative reporting career at the *New York Post* when she took an internship in her senior year of high school. She has now been there for ten years. Her work has also been featured in the *New York Times* and the *Czech Business Weekly*, where she worked when she studied abroad during her junior year of college. She was the recipient of the Silurian Award of Excellence in Journalism for Feature Writing for the article "My Mysterious Lost Month of Madness," on which this book is based. She lives in Jersey City, New Jersey.

Brain on Fire: My Month of Madness

Susannah Cahalan

Introduction

One day Susannah Cahalan woke up in a strange hospital room, strapped to her bed, under guard, and unable to move or speak. Her medical records—from a month-long hospital stay of which she had no memory—showed psychosis, violence, and dangerous instability. Yet only weeks earlier she had been a healthy, ambitious twenty-four-year-old, six months into her first serious relationship and a sparkling career as a cub reporter.

Susannah's astonishing memoir chronicles the swift path of her illness and the lucky last-minute intervention led by one of the few doctors capable of saving her life. As weeks ticked by and Susannah moved inexplicably from violence to catatonia, a million dollars worth of blood tests and brain scans revealed nothing. The exhausted doctors were ready to commit her to the psychiatric ward, in effect condemning her to a lifetime of institutions or death, until Dr. Souhel Najjar—nicknamed Dr. House— joined her team. He asked Susannah to draw one simple sketch, which became key to diagnosing her with a newly discovered autoimmune disease in which her body was attacking her brain, an illness now thought to be the cause of "demonic possessions" throughout history.

1. A quote from the philosopher Friedrich Nietzsche appears at both the beginning and end of Cahalan's memoir: "The existence of forgetting has never been proved: we only know that some things do not come to our mind when we want them to." Why do you think Cahalan chooses to recall this quotation at both the story's start and end? How does it correspond to Cahalan's tale and its major themes? In addition to the content of the quotation, why is it particularly poignant that the author would choose a quote by Nietzsche to bookend her work?

2. Evaluate and discuss the style and genre of *Brain on Fire*. Cahalan describes the book as a memoir, but she also says that it is reportage. She acknowledges using help from other sources, since she has little to no memory of many of the happenings recounted in the book. In the author's note she goes so far as to describe herself as an "unreliable source." How does this detail affect our experience of and response to her story? What does this indicate about truth and bias in storytelling? What complex issues does it raise in our understanding of works designated as nonfiction?

3. In the author's note, Cahalan says that her book is "a journalist's inquiry into that deepest part of self—personality, memory, identity." What does her story reveal about these three subjects? How does her account challenge our preconceptions of these three subjects? Alternatively, how does her account confirm or bolster what we already know and believe about these three subjects?

4. *Brain on Fire* is divided into three parts and fifty-three chapters. Why is this structure meaningful and important? How does it correspond to some of the major subjects and themes of the book? How does this structure affect our comprehension of the work or our emotional experience of it as readers?

5. Consider and discuss the various reactions to Cahalan's illness as chronicled in her book. Are the responses uni-

form or varied? Are they expected or unexpected? What about Cahalan's own responses to her illness and what she endures? Consider the response she recalls having while she was suffering versus her response after her treatment and recovery. What does consideration of these responses reveal about our responses to the mysterious and the unknown?

6. Consider and discuss your own reactions as readers to what you encounter on the page—at the opening of the story and as the story continues to its conclusion. How did your thoughts, feelings, and opinions change throughout?

7. In Chapter 22 (p. 107), Cahalan refers to a quote in William F. Allman's book *Apprentices of Wonder: Inside the Neural Network Revolution*: "The brain is a monstrous, beautiful mess." What does Allman mean by this? What does it reveal about the workings of the brain? How does this correspond to what we find revealed in Cahalan's book?

8. The characters in *Brain on Fire*—friends, family, medical personnel, and even Cahalan herself—frequently consider if she may be suffering from some form of mental illness. What does the book reveal about our way of thinking about mental illness? For instance, what does Cahalan's story suggest about the relationship between psychology and neurology? What preconceptions does it reveal about our understanding of mental illness as a society? How does this story help to highlight the necessity of compassionate responses to those who are ill?

9. Cahalan incorporates many epigraphs, quotes, and references to famous figures—Nietzsche, Aristotle, Virginia Woolf, and many others—in her story. What may be the primary reason or reasons for these being included, and why are they important?

10. Cahalan has titled her memoir *Brain on Fire*. What does this title mean and where does it come from?

11. Consider the role of faith in the story—not only religious faith, but also faith defined more broadly to include support

for others, faith in one's self (think not only of Cahalan's story but of Dr. Najjar's story), hope and resilience. What role does faith seem to play in success and recovery both for Cahalan and those around her?

12. What are some of the reasons that Cahalan may have chosen to share her story with the public? What lessons can we ultimately learn from her story?

Enhance Your Book Club

1. Write about an important experience or event in your own life. Consider how this event changed you as a person. How did others react or respond to this event? What can others learn from an account of your experience? Next, rewrite this story incorporating information from interviews of one or two people who witnessed this same event. How do the two accounts differ? How accurate is each version? Which is more believable? Does your memory of the event differ substantially from that of the subjects you interviewed? Use this exercise as a platform to initiate discussion about truth, memory, perspective, and point of view in literature.

2. Research and discuss other medical mysteries. You might consider sources such as Lisa Sanders's Diagnosis column in *The New York Times*, which inspired the hit television show *House*. What do these stories have in common with Cahalan's story? Consider and discuss your own experiences awaiting diagnosis and treatment of medical conditions. How did you and others around you react to this experience? How are these experiences like or unlike Cahalan's experience? What can we learn by considering these experiences collectively?

3. Have a film night. You might screen episodes of the Discovery Channel's *Mystery Diagnosis* or the fictional drama *House*. What connections can you draw between these mysteries and Cahalan's real-life medical mystery?

4. Read and discuss other works that challenge the mind-body connection. For instance, Malcolm's Gladwell's *Blink: The Power of Thinking Without Thinking* examines the brain's ability to instantaneously interpret information. How do such works lead us to a better understanding of ourselves and our potential? What misconceptions do these works correct? What do you find reassuring about these works? Alternatively, how are these works challenging?

5. Consider *Brain on Fire* alongside other memoirs, comparing style, narration, structure, and other formal elements. How do the works compare and how do they differ? What issues related to truth and bias in memoir surface within these stories? What do we find most compelling about these memoirs? What do these works reveal about identity, experience, and self-reflection? In addition to what we learn about the subject of each memoir, what do these books allow us to realize about others and ourselves? What does this reveal about memoir as a genre and about literature as a didactic tool?